POTS

DIET COOKBOOK FOR BEGINNERS

110+ Simple and Tasty Recipes to Manage Your Symptoms of Postural Orthostatic Tachycardia Syndrome

Kingsley Klopp

To show our appreciation for your purchase, we're delighted to offer you these special bonuses as a heartfelt thank you.

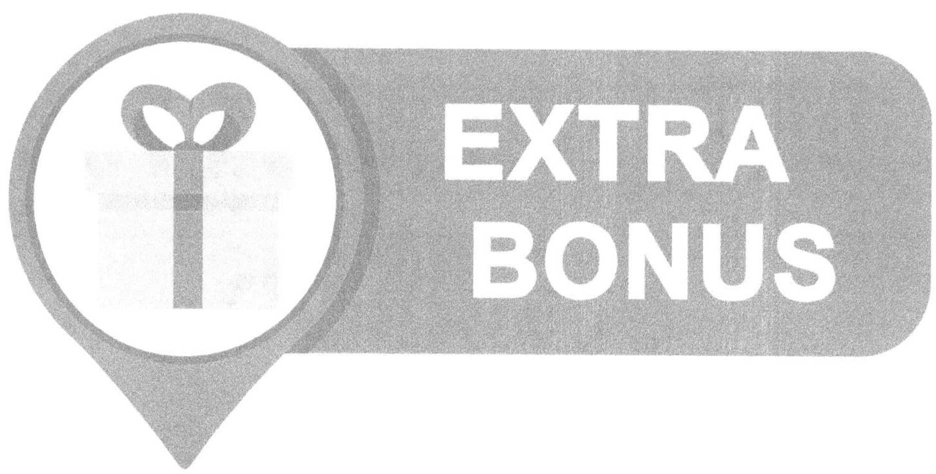

1. A Food Tracker Journal
2. Downloadable E-BOOK featuring full-color images of finished recipes

Table of Contents

Beef and Lamb Recipes

Fish and Seafood Recipes

Poultry Recipes

Soup & Stew Recipes

10-WEEK MEAL PLAN

Important Note

We are delighted to join you on this journey toward better health and symptom management through the power of nutrition. As you embark on this culinary adventure, we want to offer a gentle reminder and a few words of caution to ensure your experience is both safe and rewarding.

Every individual's body is unique, and what works wonders for one person may not be suitable for another. This is especially true for those living with Postural Orthostatic Tachycardia Syndrome (POTS). While the recipes in this book have been carefully crafted to support the nutritional needs of POTS patients, it is important to remember that individual dietary needs and tolerances can vary widely. Your personal health journey is just that—personal. Therefore, it is essential to listen to your body and adjust the recipes as needed to suit your specific circumstances. Before making any significant changes to your diet, we strongly recommend consulting with your healthcare provider. Your doctor or a registered dietitian can offer personalized advice and ensure that the dietary adjustments you make are safe and beneficial for your condition. If you encounter any confusion or uncertainty along the way, your healthcare team is there to guide you.

We also want to note that the nutritional information provided with each recipe is approximate and may vary based on the specific ingredients and brands you use. Factors such as portion sizes, ingredient substitutions, and preparation methods can influence the nutritional content of your meals. While we strive to provide accurate estimates, we encourage you to use this information as a general guide rather than an exact measure.

Our goal is to empower you with knowledge and delicious recipes that can make managing POTS a bit easier and more enjoyable. We understand the challenges you face and hope that this cookbook brings you both practical solutions and a sense of culinary delight.

Furthermore, If our cookbook has brought joy to your kitchen and table, we'd be thrilled to hear about your experiences in an Amazon review. On the flip side, if you stumble upon any hiccups while exploring our recipes, don't hesitate to get in touch at **kloppkingsley@gmail.com.** We're here to support your cooking journey every step of the way.

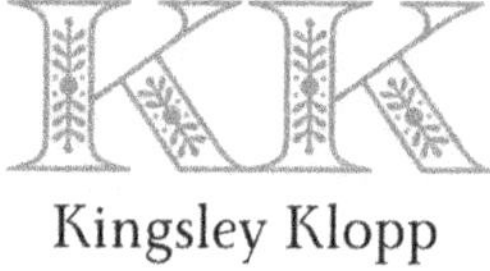

Kingsley Klopp

Introduction

Welcome to the **"POTS Diet Cookbook for Beginners"** – a comprehensive guide designed to support and nourish those living with Postural Orthostatic Tachycardia Syndrome (POTS). Whether you've recently been diagnosed or have been navigating this challenging condition for years, this book is here to be your culinary companion, offering you delicious recipes and practical advice to help manage your symptoms and improve your quality of life. Living with POTS can often feel like riding a rollercoaster with unpredictable twists and turns. One moment, you're fine, and the next, you're battling dizziness, fatigue, and a racing heart. It's a condition that can make even the simplest daily tasks seem like monumental challenges. But here's the good news: what you eat can make a significant difference in how you feel. The right diet can help stabilize your blood pressure, maintain hydration, and provide the energy you need to tackle your day with more confidence and less discomfort.

This book isn't just another cookbook. It's a thoughtfully crafted resource that blends the science of nutrition with the art of cooking, specifically tailored for the unique needs of POTS patients. We understand that managing POTS involves more than just following a list of do's and don'ts. It's about finding joy in food again, discovering meals that don't just nourish your body but also delight your taste buds. Let's start with why this book is essential. Many people with POTS struggle to find reliable dietary information that directly addresses their needs. There's a plethora of generalized dietary advice out there, but when it comes to POTS, the nuances matter. High-sodium foods, hydration strategies, nutrient-rich meals, and anti-inflammatory ingredients play crucial roles in managing symptoms. Yet, finding recipes that incorporate these elements can be daunting. That's why we've compiled a collection of recipes that are not only easy to prepare but also packed with the nutrients your body craves.

In the pages that follow, you'll find a variety of mouthwatering recipes designed to help you thrive. From hearty breakfasts that give you a strong start to your day, to satisfying lunches and dinners that keep your energy levels steady, and even snacks and desserts that are both healthy and indulgent. Each recipe has been crafted with care, ensuring they are rich in essential nutrients, balanced in flavor, and mindful of your dietary needs. But this book offers more than just recipes. It's a guide to understanding how different foods affect your body and how to make informed choices that support your health. We'll delve into the role of hydration, the importance of balanced macronutrients, and how to incorporate more high-sodium foods into your diet safely. You'll learn tips and tricks for meal planning, grocery shopping, and even dining out, making it easier to stick to your diet no matter where you are.

We know that living with POTS can be isolating and overwhelming, but you're not alone on this journey. This book is here to empower you, to give you the tools and knowledge you need to take control of your health through food. Each recipe is a step towards better management of your symptoms and a step towards reclaiming the joy of eating.

So, grab your apron, roll up your sleeves, and let's embark on this culinary adventure together. Here's to flavorful, nourishing meals that make every day a little bit brighter and every symptom a little more manageable. Welcome to the "**POTS Diet Cookbook for Beginners**" – your path to a healthier, happier you starts here.

Chapter 1: Getting Started

What is Postural Orthostatic Tachycardia Syndrome (POTS)?

Postural Orthostatic Tachycardia Syndrome (POTS) is a condition that affects the autonomic nervous system, specifically how the body regulates blood flow and blood pressure. Imagine waking up one morning, feeling dizzy and lightheaded, with your heart racing uncontrollably just from standing up. This is the daily reality for those living with POTS. It's more than just a medical condition; it's a challenging and often invisible struggle that disrupts lives and alters futures.

The Journey of POTS: From Obscurity to Recognition

The first recorded instance of what we now recognize as POTS can be traced back to the early 20th century. However, it wasn't until the 1990s that the medical community began to understand and categorize it as a distinct syndrome. Initially, patients experiencing these symptoms were often misdiagnosed with anxiety disorders, depression, or other psychological conditions. This misinterpretation led to frustration and a lack of appropriate care.

In 1993, a pivotal moment occurred when Dr. Phillip Low and Dr. Ronald Schondorf at the Mayo Clinic conducted groundbreaking research that brought clarity to this perplexing condition. They identified the specific pattern of increased heart rate upon standing without a significant drop in blood pressure, which differentiated POTS from other forms of dysautonomia. Their work was instrumental in shifting the perception of POTS from a psychological issue to a legitimate physiological disorder.

Development and Growing Awareness

Over the past few decades, awareness and understanding of POTS have grown substantially. The development of diagnostic criteria and the establishment of specialized clinics have provided much-needed support to those suffering from this condition. Organizations like Dysautonomia International have played a crucial role in advocacy, funding research, and spreading awareness.

This increased recognition has not only led to better diagnosis but also to more targeted and effective treatments. Patients now have access to a multidisciplinary approach to manage their symptoms, including lifestyle changes, medications, and physical therapy. This holistic approach can significantly improve quality of life, even if a cure remains elusive.

Living with POTS: A Daily Battle

For those affected, POTS can feel like a relentless battle against an unpredictable foe. Each day brings new challenges, from the physical symptoms to the emotional toll of living with a chronic condition. Many patients experience profound fatigue, making it difficult to maintain employment or education. The social impact can be equally isolating, as friends and family struggle to understand the invisible nature of the illness.

However, amidst the challenges, there is a resilient community of patients, caregivers, and medical professionals dedicated to improving lives. Online support groups and social media platforms have become invaluable resources for sharing experiences, advice, and encouragement. These communities offer a beacon of hope, reminding everyone affected by POTS that they are not alone in their journey.

The Future of POTS
The future holds promise for those with POTS. Research is ongoing, with scientists exploring the underlying mechanisms of the syndrome and potential new treatments. The hope is that continued advancements in medical science will lead to more effective therapies, better management strategies, and ultimately, a cure.

In the meantime, education and awareness remain crucial. By spreading knowledge about POTS, we can foster a more supportive and understanding environment for those who live with this challenging condition. Every story shared, every piece of research funded, and every new treatment developed brings us one step closer to a world where POTS no longer holds power over the lives of so many.

Symptoms and Diagnosis of POTS

Living with Postural Orthostatic Tachycardia Syndrome (POTS) can often feel like navigating a labyrinth of symptoms and uncertainties. It's a condition that can be as bewildering as it is debilitating, with a wide array of symptoms that can impact nearly every aspect of life. Understanding these symptoms and the process of diagnosis is crucial for those affected and for their loved ones who strive to support them.

The Many Faces of POTS Symptoms

POTS is characterized by a multitude of symptoms, which can vary greatly from one person to another and even from day to day for the same person. This variability makes it challenging to predict and manage, often leaving those affected feeling frustrated and misunderstood.

1. Cardiovascular Symptoms:

- Orthostatic Intolerance: The hallmark symptom of POTS is orthostatic intolerance, which means difficulty standing upright without experiencing dizziness, lightheadedness, or fainting. This happens because the body struggles to regulate blood flow and pressure when changing positions.
- Palpitations: Many people with POTS experience a rapid, pounding heartbeat when they stand up, which can be alarming and uncomfortable.
- Chest Pain: Some individuals report feeling chest pain or discomfort, which, although usually benign in the context of POTS, can be distressing and requires medical evaluation to rule out other causes.

2. Neurological Symptoms:

- Brain Fog: Cognitive impairment, often described as "brain fog," includes symptoms like difficulty concentrating, memory problems, and a general feeling of mental sluggishness.
- Headaches: Chronic headaches or migraines are common and can be severe, adding another layer of discomfort to daily life.
- Sleep Disturbances: Insomnia, poor sleep quality, and other sleep disorders frequently affect those with POTS, exacerbating fatigue and cognitive issues.

3. Gastrointestinal Symptoms:

- Nausea: Many individuals with POTS suffer from persistent nausea, which can make eating and maintaining proper nutrition challenging.
- Bloating and Pain: Abdominal bloating and pain are common, often leading to discomfort and additional digestive issues.
- Altered Bowel Movements: Diarrhea, constipation, or alternating between the two can occur, further complicating the condition.

4. Musculoskeletal Symptoms:

- Muscle Weakness: Generalized muscle weakness and fatigue can make even simple tasks feel overwhelming.
- Joint Pain: Some individuals experience joint pain, which can limit mobility and physical activity.

5. Other Symptoms:
- Temperature Regulation Issues: Difficulty regulating body temperature can lead to excessive sweating or feeling unusually cold.
- Exercise Intolerance: Physical activity often worsens symptoms, leading to an intolerance for exercise, which can complicate overall health management.
- Fatigue: Profound, debilitating fatigue is a common feature, making it hard to carry out daily activities and responsibilities.

The Diagnostic Journey

Diagnosing POTS can be a complex and often lengthy process. Many individuals go through years of seeking answers, facing misdiagnoses, and being told their symptoms are psychological. Understanding the diagnostic criteria and process can help demystify this journey and provide clarity.

1. Patient History: A detailed medical history is the first step. Physicians will ask about the onset and pattern of symptoms, any triggering events (such as a viral illness or physical trauma), and family history of similar conditions.

2. Physical Examination: A thorough physical examination helps to rule out other conditions and identify signs that may point to POTS, such as changes in heart rate and blood pressure upon standing.

3. Tilt Table Test: The tilt table test is the gold standard for diagnosing POTS. During this test, the patient is strapped to a table that tilts from a lying down to an upright position. Heart rate and blood pressure are monitored throughout. A significant increase in heart rate (at least 30 beats per minute in adults, or exceeding 120 beats per minute within 10 minutes of standing) supports a diagnosis of POTS.

4. Heart Rate and Blood Pressure Monitoring: Doctors may also use continuous heart rate and blood pressure monitoring over 24 hours to observe fluctuations and confirm the diagnosis.

5. Blood Tests: Blood tests can help rule out other conditions that might mimic POTS, such as thyroid disorders or adrenal insufficiency. They also check for markers of inflammation or other abnormalities.

6. Autonomic Function Tests: These specialized tests evaluate the autonomic nervous system's response to various stimuli, providing additional information to support the diagnosis.

7. Echocardiogram: An echocardiogram, or ultrasound of the heart, can be used to rule out structural heart problems that might contribute to symptoms.

8. QSART (Quantitative Sudomotor Axon Reflex Test): This test measures the autonomic nerves that control sweating and can provide further evidence of autonomic dysfunction.

The Role of Nutrition in POTS Management

Hydration: The Foundation of POTS Nutrition

One of the most critical aspects of nutrition for POTS patients is maintaining proper hydration. Dehydration can exacerbate symptoms such as dizziness, fatigue, and palpitations. Therefore, a key strategy in managing POTS is ensuring adequate fluid intake.

1. Increased Fluid Intake:

- Water: Drinking plenty of water throughout the day is essential. It's often recommended that individuals with POTS consume at least 2-3 liters of water daily, though this can vary based on individual needs and physician advice.
- Electrolyte Drinks: Beverages that contain electrolytes, such as sports drinks, coconut water, or specially formulated electrolyte solutions, can help maintain a balance of minerals like sodium and potassium, which are crucial for blood volume and pressure regulation.

2. Timing of Fluid Intake:

- Consistent Hydration: Rather than consuming large amounts of fluids at once, it's beneficial to drink smaller amounts consistently throughout the day to maintain stable hydration levels.
- Pre-emptive Hydration: Drinking fluids before rising in the morning or before engaging in physical activities can help mitigate the onset of symptoms.

Sodium: A Vital Component

Sodium plays a crucial role in managing POTS by helping to increase blood volume and pressure. While high sodium intake is generally discouraged in the general population, for POTS patients, it can be a necessary part of their dietary plan.

1. Increasing Sodium Intake:

- Salt Supplementation: Many POTS patients are advised to increase their salt intake, sometimes up to 3-5 grams per day, depending on individual needs and medical advice. This can be achieved through dietary sources or salt tablets.
- Salty Snacks: Incorporating salty snacks like pretzels, salted nuts, or pickles can help meet the increased sodium requirements.

2. Balanced Approach:

- Monitor Blood Pressure: Regularly monitoring blood pressure can help ensure that increased sodium intake is effective and safe.
- Consultation with Healthcare Providers: It's important to work with healthcare providers to tailor sodium intake to individual needs and avoid potential complications such as high blood pressure.

Balanced Nutrition: Ensuring Adequate Nutrient Intake

A well-balanced diet is essential for overall health and well-being, particularly for those managing a chronic condition like POTS. Ensuring adequate intake of all essential nutrients can help support energy levels, immune function, and overall health.

1. Macronutrients:

- Proteins: Lean proteins such as chicken, fish, beans, and legumes are crucial for muscle maintenance and repair, which can be beneficial given the muscle weakness and fatigue associated with POTS.
- Carbohydrates: Complex carbohydrates, such as whole grains, vegetables, and fruits, provide sustained energy release and help avoid the blood sugar spikes and crashes that can exacerbate symptoms.
- Fats: Healthy fats from sources like avocados, nuts, seeds, and olive oil are important for overall health and can help maintain energy levels.

2. Micronutrients:

- Vitamins and Minerals: Adequate intake of vitamins and minerals is essential. For example, magnesium can help with muscle function and relaxation, while potassium is important for heart health. Foods rich in these nutrients include leafy greens, nuts, seeds, and bananas.
- Iron: Given that fatigue is a significant symptom of POTS, ensuring adequate iron intake to prevent anemia is important. Iron-rich foods include red meat, spinach, and fortified cereals.

Special Dietary Considerations

Certain dietary adjustments can help manage specific symptoms and improve overall well-being for POTS patients.

1. Small, Frequent Meals:

- Avoid Large Meals: Large meals can lead to blood pooling in the digestive system, exacerbating dizziness and fatigue. Instead, smaller, more frequent meals help maintain steady blood sugar levels and energy throughout the day.

2. Low Glycemic Index Foods:

- Stabilize Blood Sugar: Foods with a low glycemic index release sugar more slowly into the bloodstream, helping to prevent spikes and crashes. Examples include whole grains, legumes, and non-starchy vegetables.

3. Avoiding Triggers:

- Identifying Food Sensitivities: Some individuals with POTS may have food sensitivities or intolerances that exacerbate symptoms. Keeping a food diary can help identify and eliminate these triggers.

4. Managing Gastrointestinal Symptoms:
- Fiber Intake: Adequate fiber intake can help manage gastrointestinal symptoms like constipation. Sources include fruits, vegetables, and whole grains.
- Probiotics: Probiotic-rich foods like yogurt and fermented vegetables can support digestive health.

Supplementation and Additional Support

While a balanced diet is the goal, some POTS patients may benefit from dietary supplements to address specific deficiencies or enhance overall nutrition.

1. Common Supplements:
- Electrolyte Supplements: These can help maintain mineral balance and hydration.
- Vitamin D and B12: These are commonly deficient in many people and can impact energy levels and overall health.
- Magnesium: Supplementation can help with muscle function and reduce cramps.

2. Professional Guidance:
- Dietitian Support: Working with a registered dietitian familiar with POTS can help tailor a nutrition plan to individual needs and ensure all dietary requirements are met.

Essential Nutrients for POTS Patients

1. Sodium: The Key Electrolyte

Importance: Sodium is vital for POTS patients because it helps increase blood volume and maintain blood pressure. Adequate sodium intake can mitigate symptoms like dizziness, lightheadedness, and fatigue.

Sources:

- Salt: Table salt is the most direct source of sodium. It can be added to meals or consumed in the form of salt tablets.
- Salty Foods: Pickles, olives, salted nuts, and pretzels are excellent snack options.
- Electrolyte Drinks: Sports drinks and specially formulated electrolyte solutions can provide a convenient source of sodium.

Recommendation: Consult with a healthcare provider to determine the appropriate daily sodium intake, which often ranges from 3-5 grams per day for POTS patients.

2. Fluids: Hydration for Stability

Importance: Staying well-hydrated is essential for maintaining blood volume and pressure, which can help reduce the severity of POTS symptoms.

Sources:

- Water: Aim for at least 2-3 liters of water daily.
- Electrolyte-Rich Beverages: Coconut water, sports drinks, and electrolyte solutions help replenish essential minerals lost through sweat.
- Herbal Teas: Caffeine-free herbal teas can contribute to daily fluid intake.

Recommendation: Drink fluids consistently throughout the day rather than consuming large amounts at once. Pre-emptive hydration, such as drinking before standing or engaging in physical activity, can also be beneficial.

3. Potassium: Balancing Sodium

Importance: Potassium works alongside sodium to regulate fluid balance, muscle contractions, and nerve signals. Adequate potassium intake is essential for cardiovascular health.

Sources:

- Fruits: Bananas, oranges, and melons are rich in potassium.
- Vegetables: Leafy greens, sweet potatoes, and avocados are excellent sources.
- Legumes: Beans, lentils, and chickpeas provide substantial potassium.

Recommendation: Include a variety of potassium-rich foods in your diet to maintain a healthy balance with sodium.

4. Magnesium: Muscle and Nerve Support

Importance: Magnesium is crucial for muscle function, nerve transmission, and maintaining a regular heartbeat. It can help reduce muscle cramps and improve overall energy levels.

Sources:

- Nuts and Seeds: Almonds, pumpkin seeds, and sunflower seeds are rich in magnesium.
- Whole Grains: Brown rice, quinoa, and oats are good sources.
- Dark Leafy Greens: Spinach and kale provide substantial magnesium.

Recommendation: Incorporate magnesium-rich foods into your diet and consider supplements if dietary intake is insufficient.

5. Vitamin D: Bone and Immune Health

Importance: Vitamin D supports bone health, immune function, and muscle strength. Many POTS patients are deficient in vitamin D, which can exacerbate symptoms.

Sources:

- Sun Exposure: The body produces vitamin D when the skin is exposed to sunlight.
- Fatty Fish: Salmon, mackerel, and sardines are rich in vitamin D.
- Fortified Foods: Milk, orange juice, and cereals often contain added vitamin D.

Recommendation: Aim for regular sun exposure and include vitamin D-rich foods in your diet. Supplements may be necessary if levels are low.

6. Iron: Preventing Anemia

Importance: Iron is essential for producing hemoglobin, which carries oxygen in the blood. Adequate iron levels can prevent anemia, a common issue that can worsen POTS symptoms like fatigue and dizziness.

Sources:

- Red Meat: Beef and lamb are rich in heme iron, which is easily absorbed by the body.
- Poultry and Fish: Chicken and fish provide good amounts of heme iron.
- Plant-Based Sources: Lentils, spinach, and fortified cereals contain non-heme iron.

Recommendation: Combine plant-based iron sources with vitamin C-rich foods to enhance absorption.

7. Vitamin B12: Energy and Nerve Function

Importance: Vitamin B12 is crucial for energy production, nerve function, and red blood cell formation. Deficiency can lead to fatigue and neurological issues.

Sources:

- Animal Products: Meat, fish, eggs, and dairy products are primary sources of vitamin B12.
- Fortified Foods: Plant-based milk and cereals often have added vitamin B12.

Recommendation: Ensure adequate intake of B12 through diet or supplements, especially if following a vegetarian or vegan diet.

8. Fiber: Digestive Health

Importance: Fiber is important for digestive health and can help manage gastrointestinal symptoms such as constipation, which is common in POTS patients.

Sources:

- Fruits and Vegetables: Apples, berries, carrots, and broccoli are high in fiber.
- Whole Grains: Oats, brown rice, and whole wheat products provide substantial fiber.
- Legumes: Beans, lentils, and chickpeas are excellent sources.

Recommendation: Include a variety of fiber-rich foods in your diet to support regular bowel movements and overall digestive health.

Hence, proper nutrition is a powerful tool in managing POTS. By focusing on essential nutrients such as sodium, potassium, magnesium, vitamin D, iron, vitamin B12, and fiber, POTS patients can significantly improve their symptoms and enhance their overall well-being. Personalized nutrition plans, developed in consultation with healthcare providers, can provide the foundation for a healthier and more manageable life with POTS.

Foods to Avoid for POTS Patients

1. High-Sugar Foods and Beverages

Why to Avoid: High-sugar foods and beverages can cause rapid spikes and subsequent crashes in blood sugar levels. These fluctuations can worsen fatigue, dizziness, and brain fog, which are already significant issues for POTS patients.

Examples:

- Sugary Snacks: Candy, cookies, pastries, and cakes.
- Sugary Beverages: Sodas, energy drinks, sweetened coffee, and tea.
- Processed Foods: Many processed foods contain hidden sugars, including sauces, dressings, and cereals.

Recommendation: Opt for whole, unprocessed foods with natural sugars, such as fruits. Read labels carefully to avoid hidden sugars.

2. Caffeinated Beverages

Why to Avoid: Caffeine can cause dehydration and increase heart rate, which can exacerbate symptoms like palpitations and anxiety. It can also lead to blood pressure fluctuations, which are problematic for POTS patients.

Examples:

- Coffee and Espresso: Regular and decaf coffee (in large amounts).
- Energy Drinks: Often high in both caffeine and sugar.
- Certain Teas: Black and green teas contain caffeine.
- Sodas: Many sodas contain caffeine, particularly colas.

Recommendation: Limit or eliminate caffeinated beverages. Herbal teas and decaf options can be good alternatives.

3. Alcohol

Why to Avoid: Alcohol can lead to dehydration and lower blood pressure, which can trigger symptoms such as dizziness, lightheadedness, and fatigue. It also impairs the body's ability to regulate blood volume and pressure.

Examples:

- Beer
- Wine
- Spirits and Liquors

Recommendation: Avoid alcohol or consume it in very limited amounts. Ensure adequate hydration if consuming alcohol.

5. High-Carbohydrate Meals

Why to Avoid: High-carbohydrate meals can cause rapid increases in blood sugar, followed by sharp drops, leading to fluctuations in energy levels and exacerbating symptoms like fatigue and brain fog.

Examples:
- White Bread and Pasta: High in refined carbohydrates.
- Pastries and Desserts: Often high in sugar and refined carbs.
- Starchy Vegetables: Large amounts of potatoes, corn, and peas.

Recommendation: Choose complex carbohydrates like whole grains and pair them with protein and healthy fats to stabilize blood sugar levels.

6. Processed and Packaged Foods

Why to Avoid: Processed foods often contain high levels of sodium, sugar, unhealthy fats, and preservatives, which can exacerbate symptoms. They also tend to lack essential nutrients needed for overall health.

Examples:
- Fast Food: High in unhealthy fats and sodium.
- Pre-Packaged Meals: Often contain preservatives and artificial ingredients.
- Snacks: Chips, crackers, and microwave popcorn.

Recommendation: Focus on whole, minimally processed foods. Prepare meals at home to control ingredients and nutrient content.

7. Artificial Sweeteners

Why to Avoid: Artificial sweeteners can cause gastrointestinal issues and may have negative effects on metabolism and blood sugar regulation, which can impact POTS symptoms.

Examples:
- Aspartame: Found in diet sodas and sugar-free products.
- Sucralose: Common in sugar-free snacks and beverages.
- Saccharin: Often used in low-calorie foods and drinks.

Recommendation: Use natural sweeteners like honey or maple syrup in moderation. Opt for whole foods that provide natural sweetness, such as fruits.

8. High-Fat Foods

Why to Avoid: High-fat foods can be difficult to digest and may lead to gastrointestinal discomfort. They can also cause blood to pool in the digestive system, exacerbating dizziness and fatigue.

Examples:
- Fried Foods: Such as french fries, fried chicken, and doughnuts.
- High-Fat Meats: Like bacon, sausage, and fatty cuts of beef.
- Full-Fat Dairy Products: Including whole milk, cream, and cheese.

Recommendation: Choose lean proteins and low-fat dairy options. Incorporate healthy fats from sources like avocados, nuts, and olive oil.

9. Foods High in Tyramine
Why to Avoid: Tyramine can affect blood pressure regulation and potentially trigger headaches and other symptoms in sensitive individuals.
Examples:
- Aged Cheeses: Such as cheddar, blue cheese, and gouda.
- Cured Meats: Including salami, pepperoni, and smoked fish.
- Fermented Foods: Such as sauerkraut, soy sauce, and certain beers.

Recommendation: Monitor intake of tyramine-rich foods and limit them if they trigger symptoms.

In conclusion understanding which foods to avoid can significantly help in managing POTS symptoms. By steering clear of high-sugar foods, caffeine, alcohol, large meals, high-carbohydrate meals, processed foods, artificial sweeteners, high-fat foods, and tyramine-rich foods, individuals with POTS can reduce symptom flare-ups and improve their overall quality of life. As always, it's essential to work with your healthcare providers to tailor dietary recommendations to individual needs and ensure a balanced, nutrient-rich diet.

Breakfast Recipes

1. Blueberry and Lemon Oatmeal

Ingredients:
- 1 cup rolled oats
- 2 cups water
- 1 cup almond milk (unsweetened)
- 1 cup fresh blueberries
- Zest of 1 lemon
- 2 tablespoons lemon juice
- 1 tablespoon chia seeds
- 1 tablespoon honey (optional)
- 1/2 teaspoon vanilla extract
- Pinch of sea salt

Instructions:
1. In a medium saucepan, combine the rolled oats, water, and almond milk.
2. Bring to a boil over medium-high heat, then reduce to a simmer.
3. Stir in the lemon zest, lemon juice, chia seeds, vanilla extract, and sea salt.
4. Cook for 5-7 minutes, stirring occasionally, until the oats are tender and the mixture has thickened.
5. Stir in the fresh blueberries and cook for an additional 2 minutes.
6. Remove from heat and drizzle with honey if desired.
7. Serve hot.

Nutrition Info (per serving):
- Calories: 220
- Carbohydrates: 40g
- Protein: 6g
- Fat: 5g
- Fiber: 8g
- Sugar: 10g

Number of Serves: 2
Cooking Time: 15 minutes

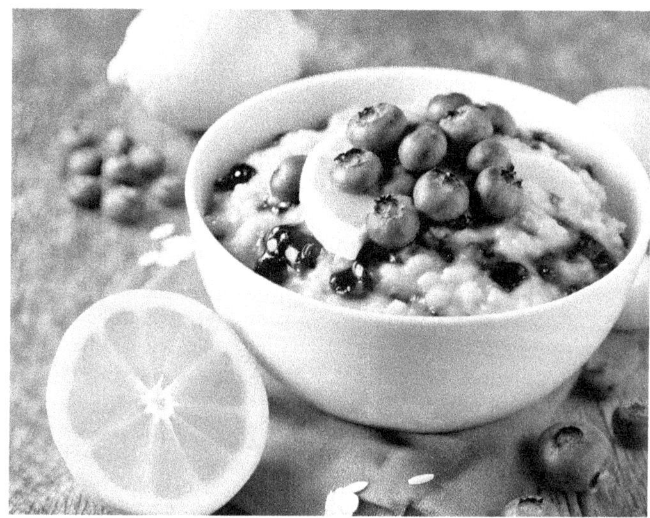

2. Cauliflower Breakfast Skillet

Ingredients:

- 2 cups cauliflower florets
- 1 small onion, diced
- 1 bell pepper, diced
- 1 small zucchini, diced
- 2 cloves garlic, minced
- 1 cup cherry tomatoes, halved
- 4 large eggs
- 1 tablespoon olive oil
- 1 teaspoon paprika
- 1/2 teaspoon turmeric
- Sea salt and pepper to taste
- Fresh parsley, chopped (for garnish)

Instructions:

1. Heat the olive oil in a large skillet over medium heat.
2. Add the onion and bell pepper, and sauté for 5 minutes until softened.
3. Add the garlic and cook for another minute.
4. Add the cauliflower florets, zucchini, and cherry tomatoes. Cook for 7-10 minutes, stirring occasionally, until the vegetables are tender.
5. Stir in the paprika, turmeric, sea salt, and pepper.
6. Create four small wells in the vegetable mixture and crack an egg into each well.
7. Cover the skillet and cook for 5-7 minutes, until the eggs are set to your liking.
8. Garnish with fresh parsley and serve immediately.

Nutrition Info (per serving):

- Calories: 200
- Carbohydrates: 12g
- Protein: 10g
- Fat: 14g
- Fiber: 4g
- Sugar: 6g

Number of Serves: 4
Cooking Time: 25 minutes

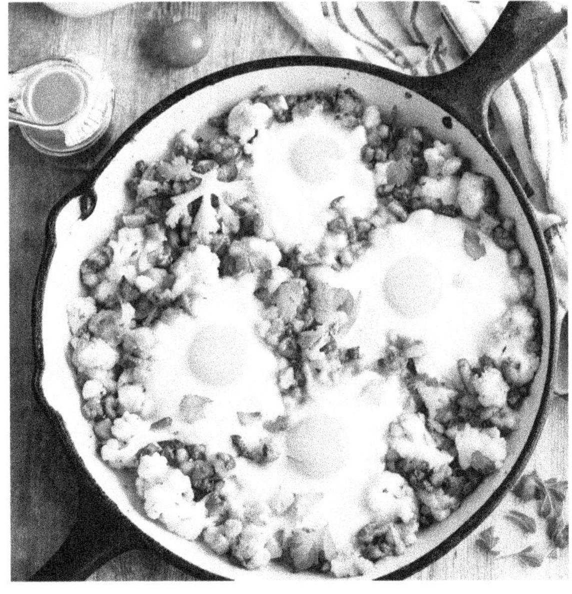

3. Hummus and Vegetable Breakfast Bowl

Ingredients:

- 1 cup cooked quinoa
- 1 cup hummus
- 1 small cucumber, diced
- 1 small carrot, grated
- 1/2 cup cherry tomatoes, halved
- 1/4 cup red cabbage, thinly sliced
- 1 avocado, sliced
- 2 tablespoons olive oil
- 1 tablespoon lemon juice
- Sea salt and pepper to taste
- Fresh parsley, chopped (for garnish)

Instructions:

1. Divide the cooked quinoa between two bowls.
2. Top each bowl with hummus, cucumber, carrot, cherry tomatoes, red cabbage, and avocado slices.
3. Drizzle with olive oil and lemon juice.
4. Season with sea salt and pepper.
5. Garnish with fresh parsley.
6. Serve immediately.

Nutrition Info (per serving):

- Calories: 350
- Carbohydrates: 40g
- Protein: 10g
- Fat: 18g
- Fiber: 12g
- Sugar: 6g

Number of Serves: 2

Cooking Time: 10 minutes

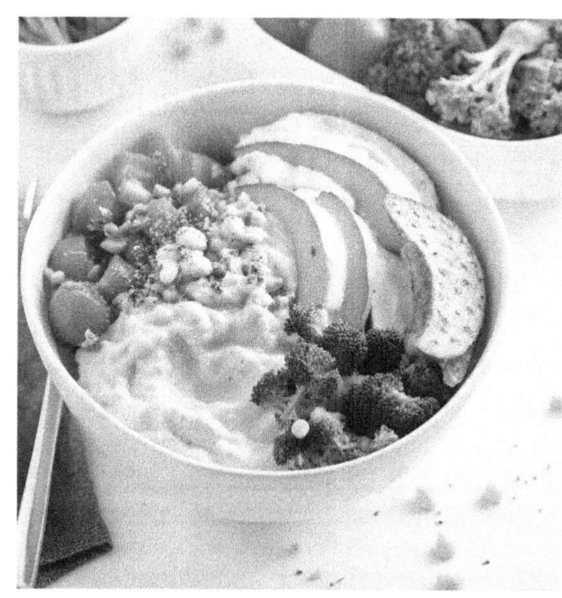

4. Overnight Oats with Chia and Flaxseeds

Ingredients:

- 1 cup rolled oats
- 1 cup almond milk (unsweetened)
- 1/2 cup Greek yogurt (optional, for added protein)
- 1 tablespoon chia seeds
- 1 tablespoon ground flaxseeds
- 1 tablespoon honey or maple syrup
- 1/2 teaspoon vanilla extract
- 1/2 cup mixed berries (fresh or frozen)

Instructions:

1. In a large bowl, combine the rolled oats, almond milk, Greek yogurt (if using), chia seeds, ground flaxseeds, honey or maple syrup, and vanilla extract.
2. Mix well to combine all ingredients.
3. Stir in the mixed berries.
4. Divide the mixture between two jars or airtight containers.
5. Cover and refrigerate overnight or for at least 4 hours.
6. In the morning, stir the oats and add a splash of almond milk if a thinner consistency is desired.
7. Serve chilled.

Nutrition Info (per serving):

- Calories: 250
- Carbohydrates: 38g
- Protein: 10g
- Fat: 8g
- Fiber: 10g
- Sugar: 12g

Number of Serves: 2

Cooking Time: 10 minutes prep, overnight refrigeration

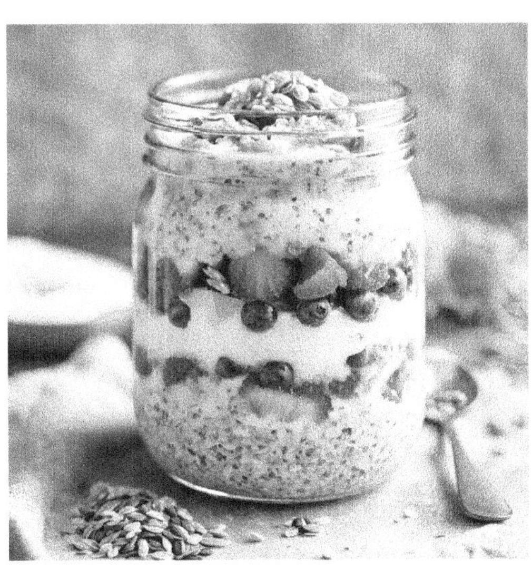

5. Soy Yogurt with Mixed Berries

Ingredients:

- 2 cups soy yogurt (unsweetened)
- 1 cup mixed berries (blueberries, strawberries, raspberries)
- 2 tablespoons chia seeds
- 1 tablespoon honey or maple syrup (optional)
- 1/2 teaspoon vanilla extract
- 1/4 cup granola (optional)

Instructions:

1. In a bowl, mix the soy yogurt with vanilla extract.
2. Divide the yogurt between two bowls.
3. Top each bowl with mixed berries.
4. Sprinkle chia seeds evenly over the top.
5. Drizzle with honey or maple syrup if desired.
6. Add granola for extra crunch, if using.
7. Serve immediately.

Nutrition Info (per serving):

- Calories: 180
- Carbohydrates: 30g
- Protein: 7g
- Fat: 4g
- Fiber: 7g
- Sugar: 12g

Number of Serves: 2
Cooking Time: 5 minutes

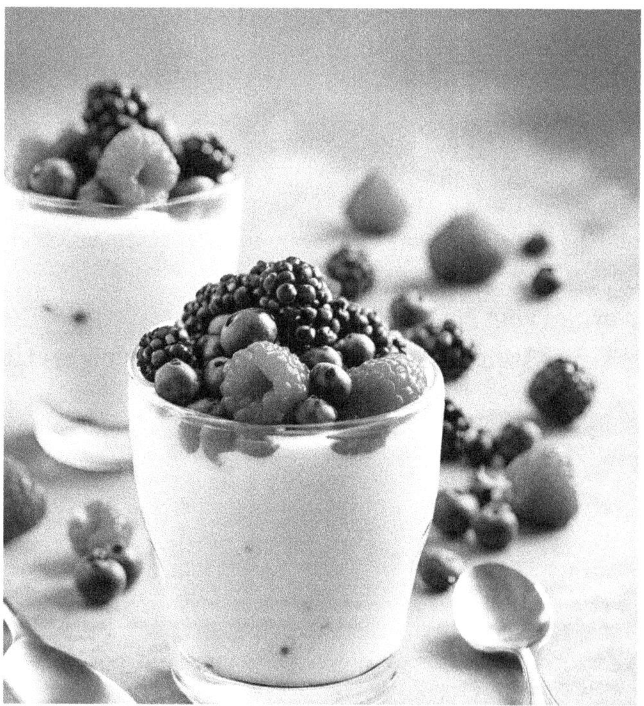

6. Cranberry Almond Breakfast Cookies

Ingredients:

- 1 cup rolled oats
- 1/2 cup almond flour
- 1/2 cup dried cranberries (unsweetened)
- 1/4 cup almond butter
- 1/4 cup honey or maple syrup
- 1 tablespoon chia seeds
- 1 tablespoon ground flaxseeds
- 1/2 teaspoon vanilla extract
- 1/4 teaspoon sea salt

Instructions:

1. Preheat the oven to 350°F (175°C) and line a baking sheet with parchment paper.
2. In a large bowl, combine rolled oats, almond flour, dried cranberries, chia seeds, ground flaxseeds, and sea salt.
3. In a separate bowl, mix almond butter, honey or maple syrup, and vanilla extract until smooth.
4. Pour the wet ingredients into the dry ingredients and mix until well combined.
5. Scoop tablespoon-sized amounts of the mixture onto the baking sheet, flattening slightly to form cookie shapes.
6. Bake for 12-15 minutes, or until the edges are golden brown.
7. Let cool on a wire rack before serving.

Nutrition Info (per serving - 1 cookie):

- Calories: 110
- Carbohydrates: 14g
- Protein: 3g
- Fat: 5g
- Fiber: 3g
- Sugar: 7g

Number of Serves: 12 cookies
Cooking Time: 20 minutes

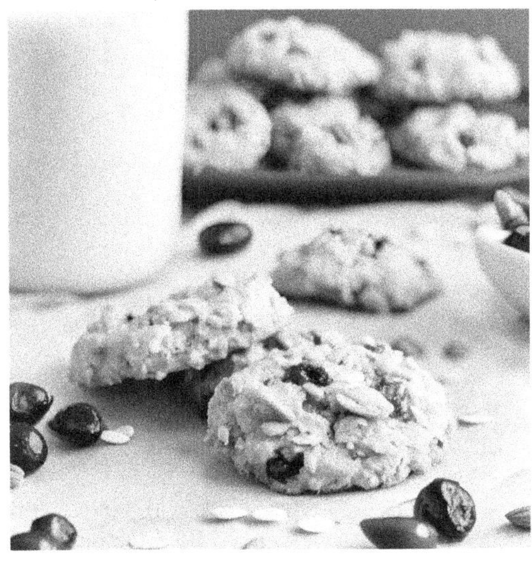

7. Spiced Lentil and Rice Porridge

Ingredients:

- 1/2 cup red lentils, rinsed
- 1/2 cup brown rice, rinsed
- 4 cups water
- 1 teaspoon ground cinnamon
- 1/2 teaspoon ground ginger
- 1/2 teaspoon turmeric
- 1/4 teaspoon sea salt
- 1 tablespoon honey or maple syrup (optional)
- 1/4 cup almond milk (unsweetened, optional)

Instructions:

1. In a large pot, combine red lentils, brown rice, and water.
2. Bring to a boil, then reduce to a simmer and cook for 25-30 minutes, or until lentils and rice are tender.
3. Stir in cinnamon, ginger, turmeric, and sea salt.
4. Cook for an additional 5 minutes, stirring occasionally.
5. Remove from heat and stir in honey or maple syrup if desired.
6. Add almond milk for a creamier texture, if desired.
7. Serve warm.

Nutrition Info (per serving):

- Calories: 200
- Carbohydrates: 38g
- Protein: 7g
- Fat: 2g
- Fiber: 7g
- Sugar: 6g

Number of Serves: 4
Cooking Time: 35 minutes

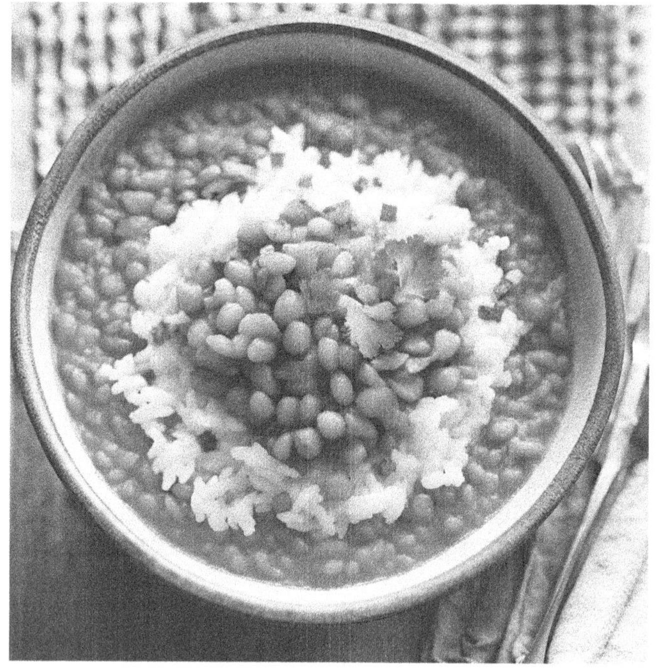

8. Maple Glazed Carrot Muffins

Ingredients:

- 1 1/2 cups whole wheat flour
- 1 teaspoon baking powder
- 1/2 teaspoon baking soda
- 1/2 teaspoon ground cinnamon
- 1/4 teaspoon ground nutmeg
- 1/4 teaspoon sea salt
- 2 cups grated carrots
- 1/2 cup unsweetened applesauce
- 1/3 cup maple syrup
- 1/4 cup almond milk (unsweetened)
- 2 tablespoons olive oil
- 1 teaspoon vanilla extract

Instructions:

1. Preheat the oven to 350°F (175°C) and line a muffin tin with paper liners.
2. In a large bowl, combine whole wheat flour, baking powder, baking soda, cinnamon, nutmeg, and sea salt.
3. In another bowl, mix grated carrots, applesauce, maple syrup, almond milk, olive oil, and vanilla extract.
4. Pour the wet ingredients into the dry ingredients and mix until just combined.
5. Divide the batter evenly among the muffin cups.
6. Bake for 20-25 minutes, or until a toothpick inserted into the center comes out clean.
7. Let cool in the tin for 5 minutes before transferring to a wire rack to cool completely.

Nutrition Info (per serving - 1 muffin):

- Calories: 150
- Carbohydrates: 24g
- Protein: 3g
- Fat: 5g
- Fiber: 4g
- Sugar: 10g

Number of Serves: 12 muffins
Cooking Time: 30 minutes

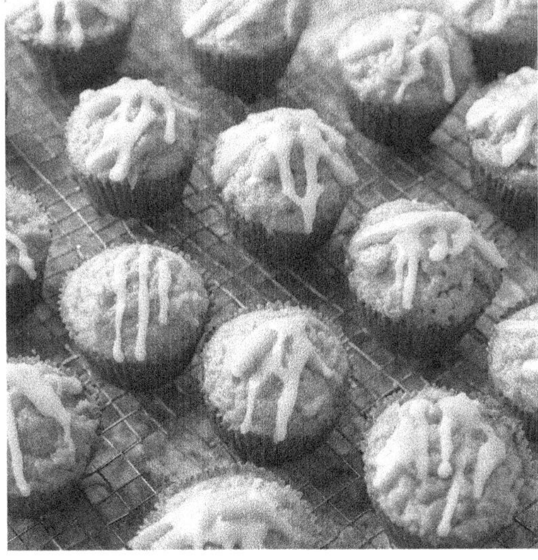

9. Vegetable and Goat Cheese Frittata

Ingredients:

- 1 tablespoon olive oil
- 1 small onion, diced
- 1 bell pepper, diced
- 1 small zucchini, diced
- 1 cup cherry tomatoes, halved
- 6 large eggs
- 1/4 cup almond milk (unsweetened)
- 1/2 cup crumbled goat cheese
- 1/4 teaspoon sea salt
- 1/4 teaspoon black pepper
- Fresh basil, chopped (for garnish)

Instructions:

1. Preheat the oven to 375°F (190°C).
2. In a large oven-safe skillet, heat the olive oil over medium heat.
3. Add the onion and bell pepper, sautéing for 5 minutes until softened.
4. Add the zucchini and cherry tomatoes, and cook for another 3-4 minutes.
5. In a bowl, whisk together the eggs, almond milk, sea salt, and black pepper.
6. Pour the egg mixture over the vegetables in the skillet.
7. Sprinkle the crumbled goat cheese evenly over the top.
8. Cook on the stovetop for 2-3 minutes until the edges begin to set.
9. Transfer the skillet to the oven and bake for 10-12 minutes, or until the frittata is set and golden.
10. Garnish with fresh basil before serving.

Nutrition Info (per serving):

- Calories: 200
- Carbohydrates: 8g
- Protein: 12g
- Fat: 14g
- Fiber: 2g
- Sugar: 5g

Number of Serves: 4

Cooking Time: 25 minutes

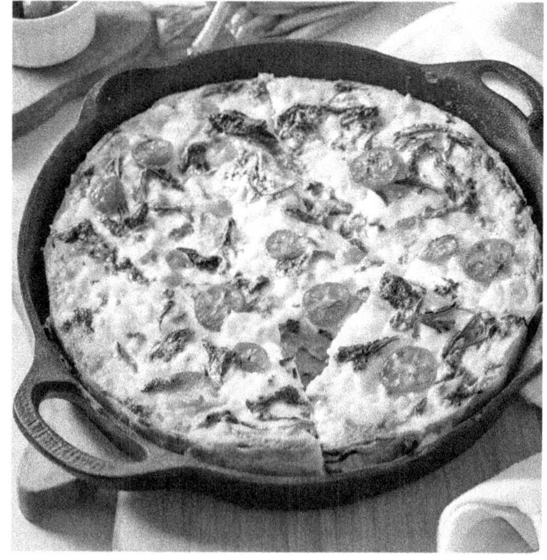

10. Mango and Lime Quinoa Salad

Ingredients:

- 1 cup quinoa, rinsed
- 2 cups water
- 1 ripe mango, diced
- 1 small red bell pepper, diced
- 1 small cucumber, diced
- 1/4 cup red onion, finely chopped
- 1/4 cup fresh cilantro, chopped
- 1/4 cup fresh lime juice (about 2 limes)
- 1 tablespoon olive oil
- 1 teaspoon honey or maple syrup (optional)
- Sea salt and pepper to taste

Instructions:

1. In a medium saucepan, combine the quinoa and water. Bring to a boil, then reduce to a simmer and cook for 15 minutes, or until the quinoa is tender and water is absorbed.
2. Remove from heat and let cool.
3. In a large bowl, combine the cooked quinoa, mango, bell pepper, cucumber, red onion, and cilantro.
4. In a small bowl, whisk together the lime juice, olive oil, honey or maple syrup (if using), sea salt, and pepper.
5. Pour the dressing over the quinoa mixture and toss to combine.
6. Serve chilled or at room temperature.

Nutrition Info (per serving):

- Calories: 250
- Carbohydrates: 42g
- Protein: 6g
- Fat: 7g
- Fiber: 6g
- Sugar: 15g

Number of Serves: 4
Cooking Time: 20 minutes

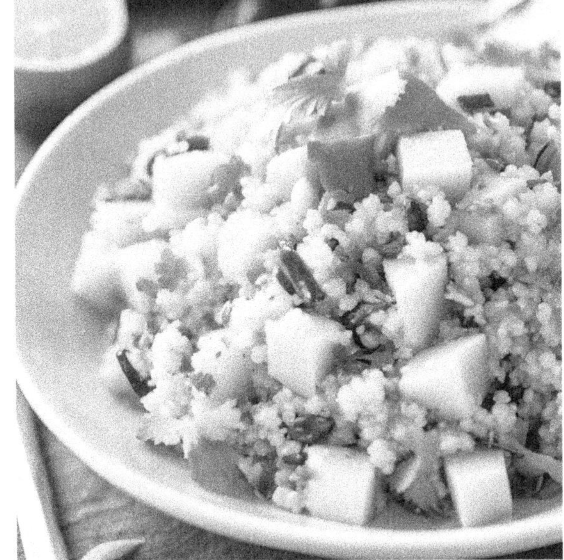

11. Protein-Packed Breakfast Bars

Ingredients:

- 1 1/2 cups rolled oats
- 1/2 cup almond flour
- 1/2 cup almond butter
- 1/4 cup honey or maple syrup
- 1/4 cup unsweetened dried cranberries
- 1/4 cup sunflower seeds
- 1/4 cup pumpkin seeds
- 2 tablespoons chia seeds
- 1 teaspoon vanilla extract
- 1/4 teaspoon sea salt

Instructions:

1. Preheat the oven to 350°F (175°C) and line an 8x8-inch baking dish with parchment paper.
2. In a large bowl, mix together the rolled oats, almond flour, dried cranberries, sunflower seeds, pumpkin seeds, chia seeds, and sea salt.
3. In a separate bowl, combine the almond butter, honey or maple syrup, and vanilla extract until smooth.
4. Pour the wet ingredients into the dry ingredients and mix until well combined.
5. Press the mixture evenly into the prepared baking dish.
6. Bake for 20-25 minutes, or until the edges are golden brown.
7. Let cool completely before cutting into bars.

Nutrition Info (per serving):

- Calories: 220
- Carbohydrates: 26g
- Protein: 6g
- Fat: 11g
- Fiber: 5g
- Sugar: 10g

Number of Serves: 12 bars

Cooking Time: 30 minutes

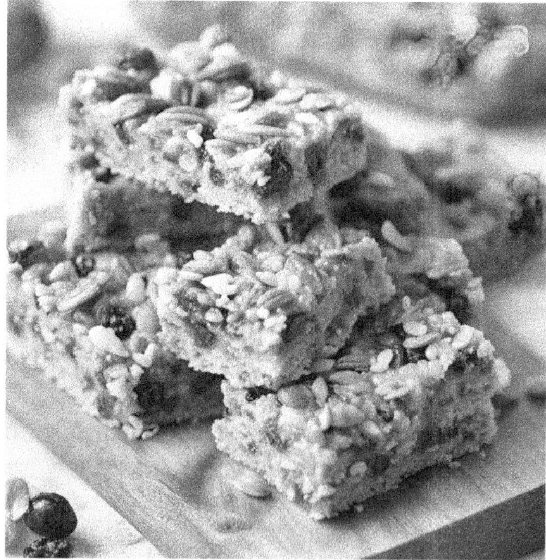

12. Almond Butter and Banana Sandwich

Ingredients:

- 2 slices whole grain bread
- 2 tablespoons almond butter
- 1 banana, sliced
- 1 tablespoon chia seeds
- 1/2 teaspoon honey (optional)

Instructions:

1. Toast the slices of whole grain bread until golden brown.
2. Spread almond butter evenly on one side of each slice of bread.
3. Arrange banana slices on one slice of bread.
4. Sprinkle chia seeds over the banana slices.
5. Drizzle with honey if desired.
6. Top with the second slice of bread, almond butter side down.
7. Cut in half and serve immediately.

Nutrition Info (per serving):

- Calories: 300
- Carbohydrates: 40g
- Protein: 9g
- Fat: 14g
- Fiber: 8g
- Sugar: 12g

Number of Serves: 1
Cooking Time: 5 minutes

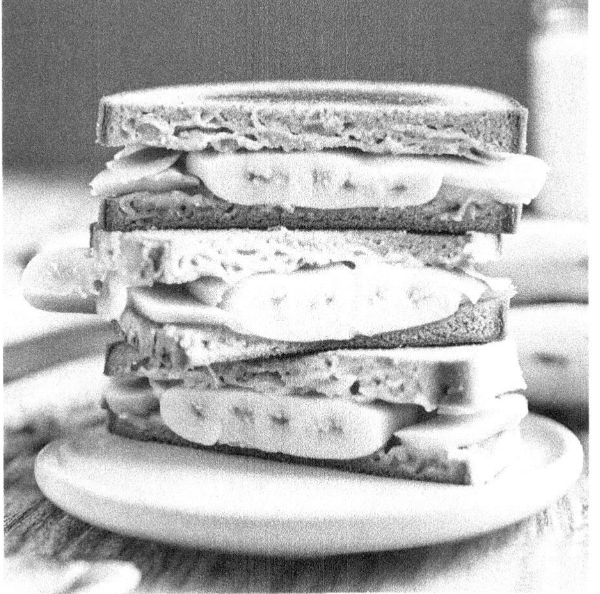

13. Kale and Potato Breakfast Hash

Ingredients:

- 2 tablespoons olive oil
- 1 small onion, diced
- 2 cloves garlic, minced
- 2 medium potatoes, diced
- 1 cup chopped kale
- 1/2 teaspoon paprika
- 1/2 teaspoon sea salt
- 1/4 teaspoon black pepper
- 4 large eggs
- Fresh parsley, chopped (for garnish)

Instructions:

1. Heat olive oil in a large skillet over medium heat.
2. Add the onion and garlic, sautéing for 3-4 minutes until softened.
3. Add the diced potatoes and cook for 10-12 minutes, stirring occasionally, until golden and tender.
4. Stir in the chopped kale, paprika, sea salt, and black pepper. Cook for an additional 3-4 minutes until the kale is wilted.
5. Create four small wells in the hash and crack an egg into each well.
6. Cover the skillet and cook for 5-7 minutes, until the eggs are set to your liking.
7. Garnish with fresh parsley and serve immediately.

Nutrition Info (per serving):

- Calories: 250
- Carbohydrates: 20g
- Protein: 10g
- Fat: 15g
- Fiber: 4g
- Sugar: 3g

Number of Serves: 4

Cooking Time: 25 minutes

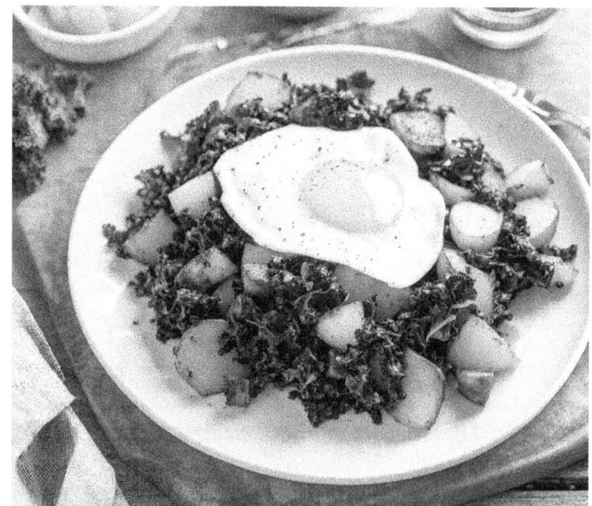

14. Buckwheat Pancakes

Ingredients:

- 1 cup buckwheat flour
- 1 teaspoon baking powder
- 1/2 teaspoon baking soda
- 1/4 teaspoon sea salt
- 1 cup almond milk (unsweetened)
- 1 large egg
- 2 tablespoons maple syrup
- 1 teaspoon vanilla extract
- 2 tablespoons olive oil (for cooking)

Instructions:

1. In a large bowl, whisk together the buckwheat flour, baking powder, baking soda, and sea salt.
2. In another bowl, mix the almond milk, egg, maple syrup, and vanilla extract until well combined.
3. Pour the wet ingredients into the dry ingredients and mix until just combined.
4. Heat a non-stick skillet over medium heat and add a little olive oil.
5. Pour 1/4 cup of batter onto the skillet for each pancake.
6. Cook until bubbles form on the surface, then flip and cook until golden brown on the other side, about 2-3 minutes per side.
7. Repeat with the remaining batter, adding more oil as needed.
8. Serve with additional maple syrup if desired.

Nutrition Info (per serving):

- Calories: 120
- Carbohydrates: 18g
- Protein: 4g
- Fat: 4g
- Fiber: 3g
- Sugar: 3g

Number of Serves: 4
Cooking Time: 20 minutes

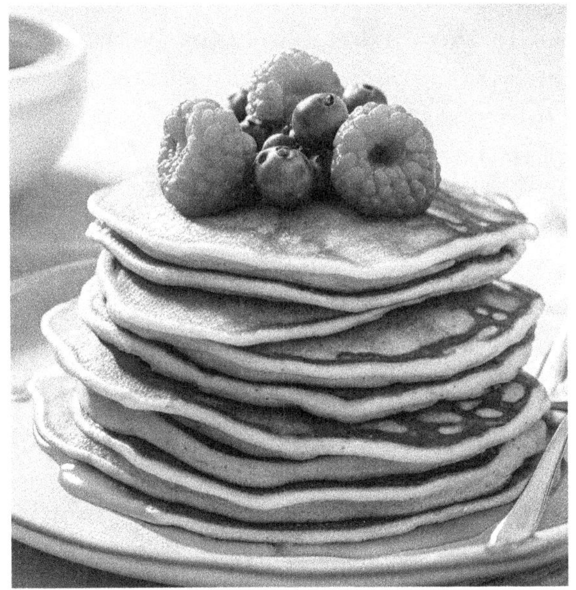

15. Raspberry Almond Muffins

Ingredients:

- 1 1/2 cups almond flour
- 1/2 cup rolled oats
- 1 teaspoon baking powder
- 1/2 teaspoon baking soda
- 1/4 teaspoon sea salt
- 1/2 cup unsweetened applesauce
- 1/4 cup almond milk (unsweetened)
- 1/4 cup honey or maple syrup
- 1 teaspoon vanilla extract
- 1 cup fresh raspberries
- 1/4 cup sliced almonds

Instructions:

1. Preheat the oven to 350°F (175°C) and line a muffin tin with paper liners.
2. In a large bowl, combine almond flour, rolled oats, baking powder, baking soda, and sea salt.
3. In another bowl, mix applesauce, almond milk, honey or maple syrup, and vanilla extract until well combined.
4. Pour the wet ingredients into the dry ingredients and mix until just combined.
5. Gently fold in the fresh raspberries.
6. Divide the batter evenly among the muffin cups and sprinkle with sliced almonds.
7. Bake for 20-25 minutes, or until a toothpick inserted into the center comes out clean.
8. Let cool in the tin for 5 minutes before transferring to a wire rack to cool completely.

Nutrition Info (per serving - 1 muffin):

- Calories: 140
- Carbohydrates: 20g
- Protein: 4g
- Fat: 7g
- Fiber: 4g
- Sugar: 8g

Number of Serves: 12 muffins

Cooking Time: 30 minutes

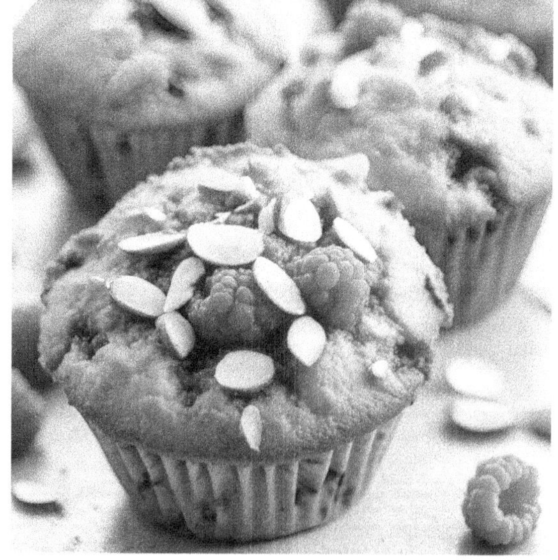

16. Tofu Scramble

Ingredients:

- 1 tablespoon olive oil
- 1 small onion, diced
- 1 bell pepper, diced
- 2 cloves garlic, minced
- 1 block (14 oz) firm tofu, drained and crumbled
- 1 teaspoon ground turmeric
- 1/2 teaspoon ground cumin
- 1/2 teaspoon paprika
- 1/4 teaspoon sea salt
- 1/4 teaspoon black pepper
- 1 cup baby spinach
- Fresh cilantro, chopped (for garnish)

Instructions:

1. Heat the olive oil in a large skillet over medium heat.
2. Add the onion and bell pepper, sautéing for 5 minutes until softened.
3. Add the garlic and cook for another minute.
4. Stir in the crumbled tofu, turmeric, cumin, paprika, sea salt, and black pepper. Cook for 5-7 minutes, stirring occasionally, until the tofu is heated through and evenly coated with spices.
5. Add the baby spinach and cook for another 2-3 minutes until wilted.
6. Garnish with fresh cilantro and serve immediately.

Nutrition Info (per serving):

- Calories: 180
- Carbohydrates: 10g
- Protein: 15g
- Fat: 10g
- Fiber: 4g
- Sugar: 3g

Number of Serves: 4
Cooking Time: 20 minutes

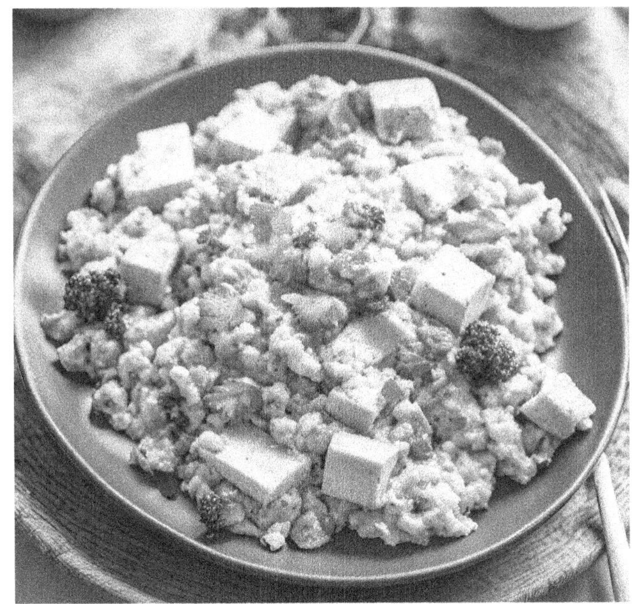

17. Baked Pears with Walnuts and Honey

Ingredients:

- 4 ripe pears, halved and cored
- 1/2 cup walnuts, chopped
- 2 tablespoons honey
- 1 teaspoon ground cinnamon
- 1/4 teaspoon ground nutmeg
- 1/4 cup water
- Fresh mint leaves (for garnish, optional)

Instructions:

1. Preheat the oven to 350°F (175°C).
2. Place the pear halves cut side up in a baking dish.
3. In a small bowl, mix the chopped walnuts, honey, cinnamon, and nutmeg.
4. Spoon the walnut mixture into the hollowed centers of the pears.
5. Pour the water into the baking dish to cover the bottom.
6. Bake for 25-30 minutes, or until the pears are tender.
7. Remove from the oven and let cool slightly.
8. Garnish with fresh mint leaves if desired and serve warm.

Nutrition Info (per serving):

- Calories: 160
- Carbohydrates: 30g
- Protein: 2g
- Fat: 6g
- Fiber: 5g
- Sugar: 22g

Number of Serves: 4

Cooking Time: 35 minutes

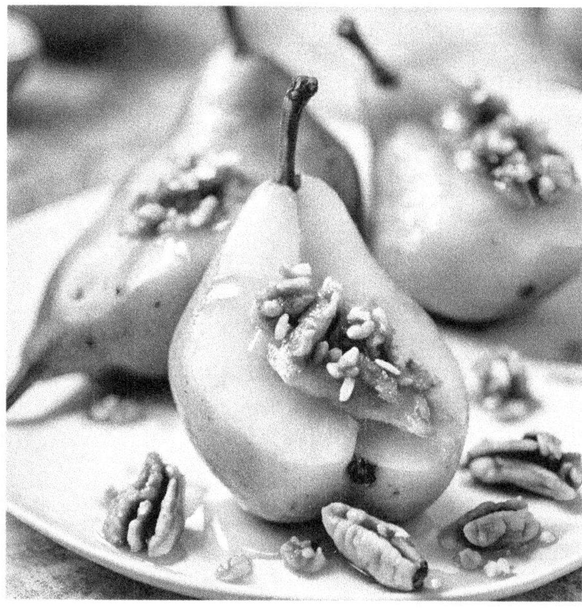

18. Pumpkin Spice Smoothie

Ingredients:

- 1 cup pumpkin puree
- 1 ripe banana
- 1 cup almond milk (unsweetened)
- 1/2 cup Greek yogurt (optional, for added protein)
- 1 tablespoon chia seeds
- 1 tablespoon honey or maple syrup
- 1/2 teaspoon ground cinnamon
- 1/4 teaspoon ground nutmeg
- 1/4 teaspoon ground ginger
- 1/4 teaspoon ground cloves
- 1/2 teaspoon vanilla extract
- Ice cubes (optional)

Instructions:

1. Combine the pumpkin puree, banana, almond milk, Greek yogurt (if using), chia seeds, honey or maple syrup, cinnamon, nutmeg, ginger, cloves, and vanilla extract in a blender.
2. Blend until smooth.
3. Add ice cubes if desired and blend again until smooth.
4. Pour into glasses and serve immediately.

Nutrition Info (per serving):

- Calories: 220
- Carbohydrates: 40g
- Protein: 7g
- Fat: 4g
- Fiber: 8g
- Sugar: 22g

Number of Serves: 2

Cooking Time: 5 minutes

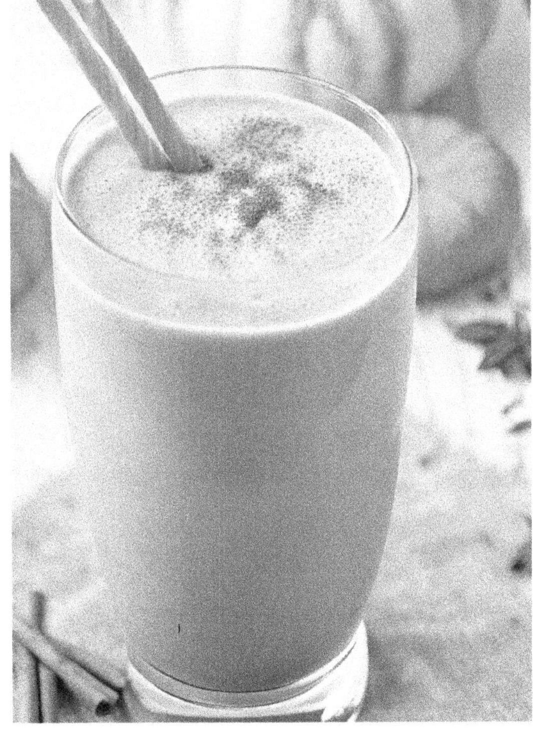

19. Quinoa Porridge

Ingredients:

- 1 cup quinoa, rinsed
- 2 cups water
- 1 cup almond milk (unsweetened)
- 1 tablespoon honey or maple syrup
- 1 teaspoon ground cinnamon
- 1/4 teaspoon sea salt
- 1/2 teaspoon vanilla extract
- 1/2 cup fresh berries (optional, for topping)
- 1/4 cup chopped nuts (optional, for topping)

Instructions:

1. In a medium saucepan, combine the quinoa and water. Bring to a boil, then reduce to a simmer and cook for 15 minutes, or until the quinoa is tender and water is absorbed.
2. Add the almond milk, honey or maple syrup, cinnamon, sea salt, and vanilla extract. Stir to combine.
3. Cook for an additional 5-7 minutes, stirring frequently, until the porridge reaches the desired consistency.
4. Serve topped with fresh berries and chopped nuts if desired.

Nutrition Info (per serving):

- Calories: 240
- Carbohydrates: 40g
- Protein: 7g
- Fat: 7g
- Fiber: 5g
- Sugar: 10g

Number of Serves: 4
Cooking Time: 25 minutes

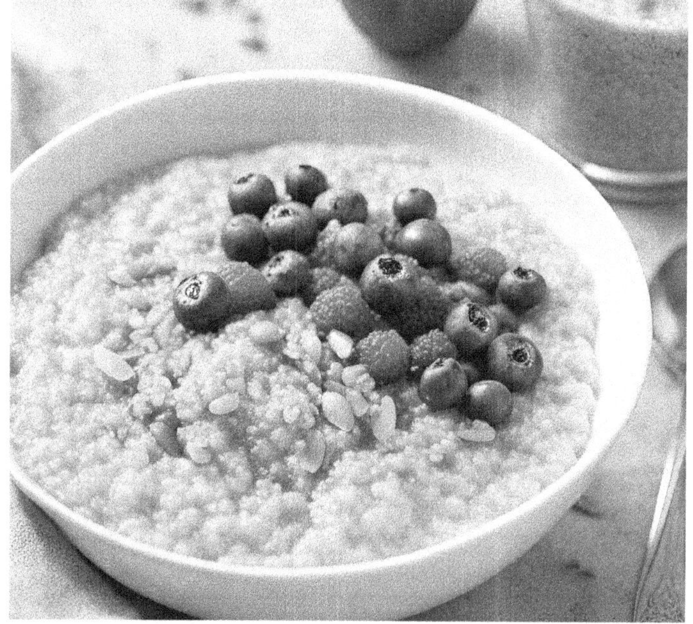

20. Spinach and Feta Omelette

Ingredients:

- 1 tablespoon olive oil
- 1 small onion, diced
- 2 cups fresh spinach, chopped
- 4 large eggs
- 1/4 cup almond milk (unsweetened)
- 1/2 cup crumbled feta cheese
- 1/4 teaspoon sea salt
- 1/4 teaspoon black pepper
- Fresh parsley, chopped (for garnish)

Instructions:

1. Heat the olive oil in a large non-stick skillet over medium heat.
2. Add the diced onion and sauté for 3-4 minutes until softened.
3. Add the chopped spinach and cook for another 2-3 minutes until wilted.
4. In a bowl, whisk together the eggs, almond milk, sea salt, and black pepper.
5. Pour the egg mixture over the vegetables in the skillet.
6. Cook until the edges start to set, then sprinkle the crumbled feta cheese over the top.
7. Cover the skillet and cook for 3-5 minutes, or until the omelette is fully set and the cheese is melted.
8. Garnish with fresh parsley and serve immediately.

Nutrition Info (per serving):

- Calories: 220
- Carbohydrates: 6g
- Protein: 14g
- Fat: 16g
- Fiber: 2g
- Sugar: 3g

Number of Serves: 2
Cooking Time: 15 minutes

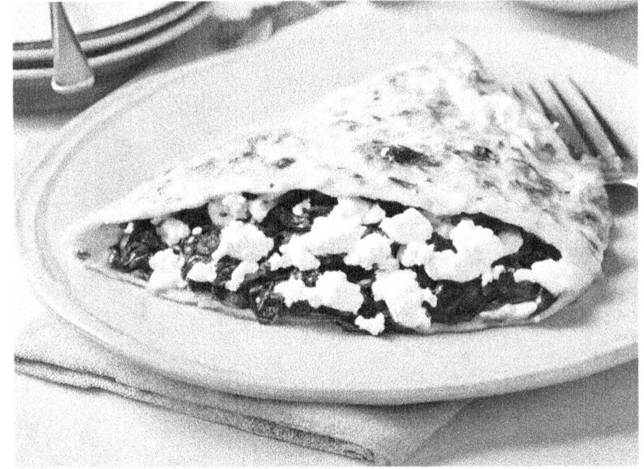

21. Chicken Sausage and Sweet Potato Hash

Ingredients:

- 1 tablespoon olive oil
- 1 small onion, diced
- 2 cloves garlic, minced
- 2 medium sweet potatoes, peeled and diced
- 4 chicken sausages, sliced
- 1 red bell pepper, diced
- 1 green bell pepper, diced
- 1 teaspoon paprika
- 1/2 teaspoon sea salt
- 1/4 teaspoon black pepper
- Fresh parsley, chopped (for garnish)

Instructions:

1. Heat the olive oil in a large skillet over medium heat.
2. Add the diced onion and garlic, sautéing for 3-4 minutes until softened.
3. Add the sweet potatoes and cook for 10-12 minutes, stirring occasionally, until tender.
4. Add the sliced chicken sausages, red bell pepper, and green bell pepper to the skillet. Cook for an additional 5-7 minutes, until the vegetables are tender and the sausage is cooked through.
5. Stir in the paprika, sea salt, and black pepper.
6. Garnish with fresh parsley before serving.

Nutrition Info (per serving):

- Calories: 300
- Carbohydrates: 30g
- Protein: 15g
- Fat: 15g
- Fiber: 6g
- Sugar: 8g

Number of Serves: 4
Cooking Time: 25 minutes

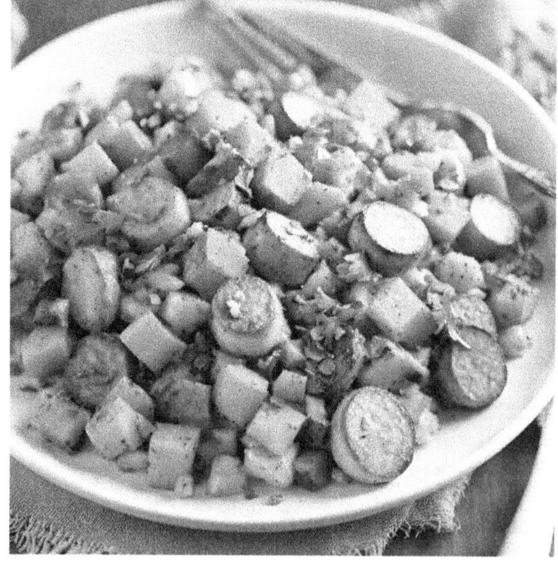

22. Salted Peanut Butter Oatmeal

Ingredients:

- 1 cup rolled oats
- 2 cups water
- 1 cup almond milk (unsweetened)
- 2 tablespoons peanut butter (unsweetened)
- 1 tablespoon honey or maple syrup
- 1/4 teaspoon sea salt
- 1/2 teaspoon vanilla extract
- 1/4 cup crushed peanuts (optional, for topping)

Instructions:

1. In a medium saucepan, combine the rolled oats, water, and almond milk. Bring to a boil, then reduce to a simmer.
2. Cook for 5-7 minutes, stirring occasionally, until the oats are tender and the mixture has thickened.
3. Stir in the peanut butter, honey or maple syrup, sea salt, and vanilla extract until well combined.
4. Serve hot, topped with crushed peanuts if desired.

Nutrition Info (per serving):

- Calories: 280
- Carbohydrates: 40g
- Protein: 8g
- Fat: 10g
- Fiber: 6g
- Sugar: 12g

Number of Serves: 2
Cooking Time: 10 minutes

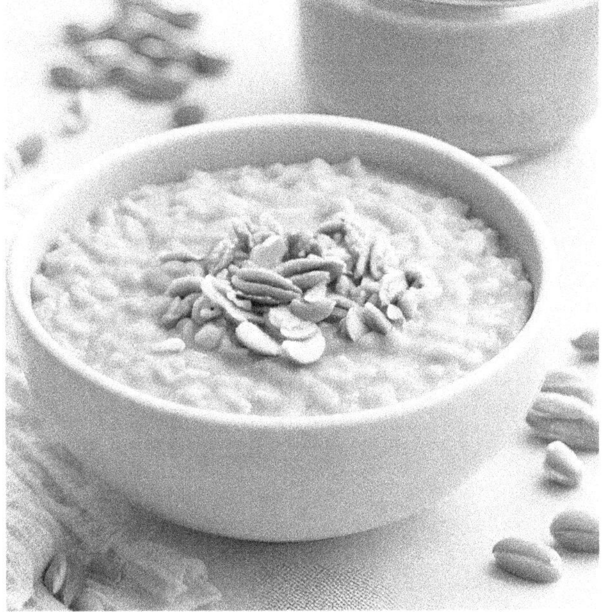

23. Egg Muffins

Ingredients:

- 8 large eggs
- 1/2 cup almond milk (unsweetened)
- 1 cup diced vegetables (bell peppers, spinach, onions)
- 1/2 cup shredded cheese (optional)
- 1/2 teaspoon sea salt
- 1/4 teaspoon black pepper
- 1/2 teaspoon paprika
- Olive oil spray (for greasing)

Instructions:

1. Preheat the oven to 350°F (175°C) and grease a muffin tin with olive oil spray.
2. In a large bowl, whisk together the eggs, almond milk, sea salt, black pepper, and paprika.
3. Stir in the diced vegetables and shredded cheese (if using).
4. Pour the egg mixture evenly into the muffin tin cups.
5. Bake for 20-25 minutes, or until the egg muffins are set and lightly golden.
6. Let cool slightly before removing from the tin.

Nutrition Info (per serving - 1 muffin):

- Calories: 80
- Carbohydrates: 2g
- Protein: 6g
- Fat: 5g
- Fiber: 1g
- Sugar: 1g

Number of Serves: 12 muffins

Cooking Time: 30 minutes

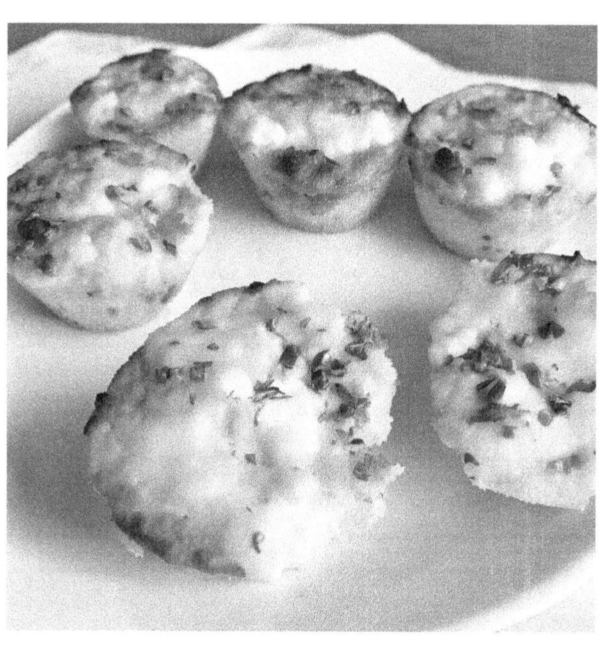

24. Greek Yogurt Parfait

Ingredients:

- 2 cups Greek yogurt (unsweetened)
- 1 cup mixed berries (blueberries, strawberries, raspberries)
- 1/4 cup granola (optional)
- 2 tablespoons chia seeds
- 1 tablespoon honey or maple syrup

Instructions:

1. In two serving glasses, layer the Greek yogurt and mixed berries.
2. Sprinkle chia seeds and granola (if using) between the layers.
3. Drizzle honey or maple syrup over the top.
4. Serve immediately.

Nutrition Info (per serving):

- Calories: 200
- Carbohydrates: 25g
- Protein: 12g
- Fat: 6g
- Fiber: 6g
- Sugar: 18g

Number of Serves: 2
Cooking Time: 5 minutes

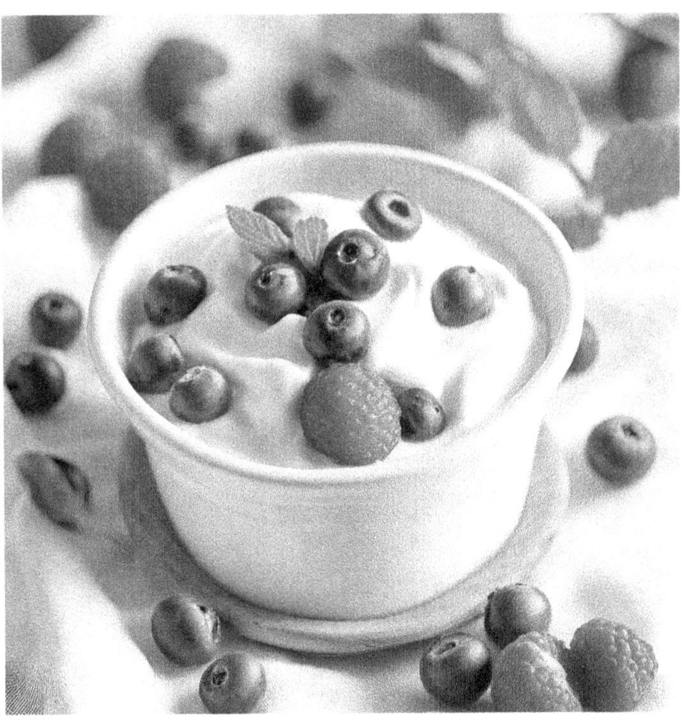

25. Banana Oatmeal Pancakes

Ingredients:

- 1 cup rolled oats
- 1 ripe banana
- 2 large eggs
- 1/4 cup almond milk (unsweetened)
- 1 teaspoon baking powder
- 1/2 teaspoon vanilla extract
- Olive oil spray (for cooking)

Instructions:

1. In a blender, combine the rolled oats, banana, eggs, almond milk, baking powder, and vanilla extract. Blend until smooth.
2. Heat a non-stick skillet over medium heat and spray with olive oil.
3. Pour 1/4 cup of batter onto the skillet for each pancake.
4. Cook until bubbles form on the surface, then flip and cook until golden brown on the other side, about 2-3 minutes per side.
5. Repeat with the remaining batter, adding more oil as needed.
6. Serve warm with your favorite toppings.

Nutrition Info (per serving):

- Calories: 120
- Carbohydrates: 18g
- Protein: 5g
- Fat: 4g
- Fiber: 3g
- Sugar: 6g

Number of Serves: 4
Cooking Time: 20 minutes

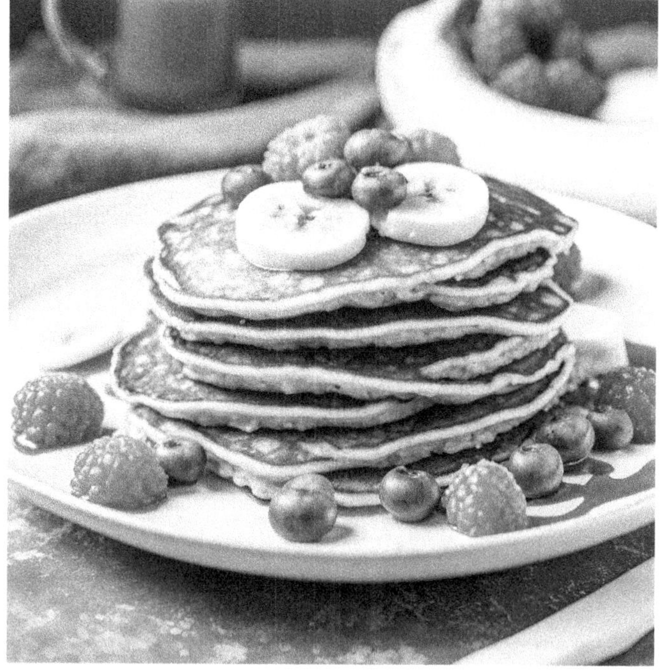

Beef and Lamb Recipes

1. Beef Stir-Fry with Broccoli and Bell Peppers
Ingredients:
- 1 lb beef sirloin, thinly sliced
- 2 cups broccoli florets
- 1 red bell pepper, thinly sliced
- 1 yellow bell pepper, thinly sliced
- 1 small onion, thinly sliced
- 3 cloves garlic, minced
- 1 tablespoon ginger, minced
- 3 tablespoons soy sauce (low sodium)
- 2 tablespoons olive oil
- 1 tablespoon cornstarch
- 1/4 cup water
- 1 tablespoon sesame oil (optional)
- 1/4 teaspoon sea salt
- 1/4 teaspoon black pepper
- Cooked brown rice, for serving

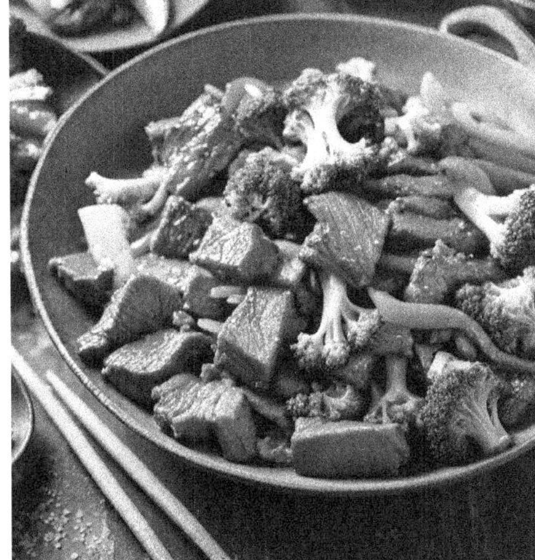

Instructions:
1. In a small bowl, mix the soy sauce, cornstarch, and water. Set aside.
2. Heat 1 tablespoon of olive oil in a large skillet over medium-high heat.
3. Add the sliced beef, sea salt, and black pepper, cooking until browned and cooked through, about 4-5 minutes. Remove from the skillet and set aside.
4. In the same skillet, add the remaining tablespoon of olive oil.
5. Add the onion, garlic, and ginger, sautéing for 2-3 minutes until fragrant.
6. Add the broccoli and bell peppers, cooking for another 5-7 minutes until tender.
7. Return the beef to the skillet and pour in the soy sauce mixture.
8. Cook for an additional 2-3 minutes until the sauce has thickened.
9. Drizzle with sesame oil if desired.
10. Serve hot over cooked brown rice.

Nutrition Info (per serving):
- Calories: 320
- Carbohydrates: 22g
- Protein: 28g
- Fat: 14g
- Fiber: 5g
- Sugar: 6g

Number of Serves: 4
Cooking Time: 20 minutes

2. Classic Beef Stew

Ingredients:

- 1 1/2 lbs beef chuck, cut into 1-inch cubes
- 2 tablespoons olive oil
- 1 large onion, diced
- 3 cloves garlic, minced
- 4 cups beef broth (low sodium)
- 2 cups water
- 3 large carrots, peeled and sliced
- 3 medium potatoes, peeled and diced
- 2 celery stalks, sliced
- 2 tablespoons tomato paste
- 1 teaspoon dried thyme
- 1 teaspoon dried rosemary
- 1 bay leaf
- 1/4 teaspoon sea salt
- 1/4 teaspoon black pepper
- 2 tablespoons cornstarch (optional, for thickening)

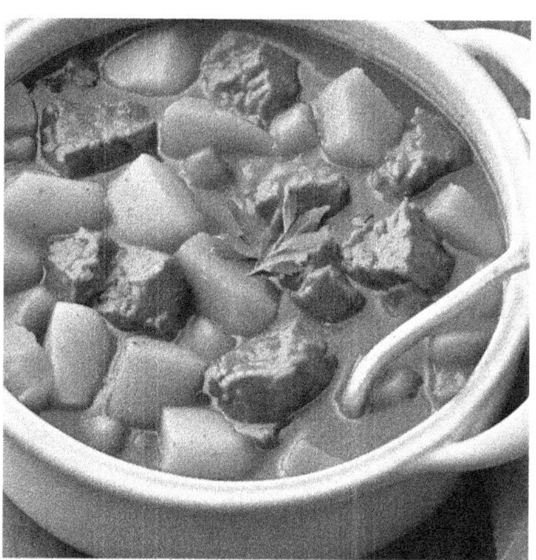

Instructions:

1. Heat the olive oil in a large pot over medium-high heat.
2. Add the beef cubes, sea salt, and black pepper, browning on all sides, about 5-7 minutes. Remove and set aside.
3. In the same pot, add the onion and garlic, sautéing for 3-4 minutes until softened.
4. Stir in the tomato paste and cook for another minute.
5. Add the beef broth, water, browned beef, carrots, potatoes, celery, thyme, rosemary, and bay leaf.
6. Bring to a boil, then reduce heat to low and simmer for 1 1/2 to 2 hours, or until the beef is tender.
7. If a thicker stew is desired, mix the cornstarch with a little water to form a slurry and stir it into the stew during the last 10 minutes of cooking.
8. Remove the bay leaf before serving.
9. Serve hot.

Nutrition Info (per serving):

- Calories: 350
- Carbohydrates: 30g
- Protein: 28g
- Fat: 12g
- Fiber: 5g
- Sugar: 6g

Number of Serves: 6

Cooking Time: 2 hours

3. Grilled Lamb Chops with Mint Yogurt

Ingredients:

- 8 lamb chops
- 2 tablespoons olive oil
- 2 cloves garlic, minced
- 1 tablespoon fresh rosemary, chopped
- 1/2 teaspoon sea salt
- 1/2 teaspoon black pepper
- 1 cup Greek yogurt (unsweetened)
- 1/4 cup fresh mint, chopped
- 1 tablespoon lemon juice
- 1/2 teaspoon honey or maple syrup

Instructions:

1. In a small bowl, mix the olive oil, garlic, rosemary, sea salt, and black pepper.
2. Rub the mixture evenly over the lamb chops.
3. Preheat the grill to medium-high heat.
4. Grill the lamb chops for 3-4 minutes per side for medium-rare, or until the desired doneness is reached.
5. In a separate bowl, combine the Greek yogurt, fresh mint, lemon juice, and honey or maple syrup.
6. Serve the grilled lamb chops with the mint yogurt sauce on the side.

Nutrition Info (per serving):

- Calories: 380
- Carbohydrates: 6g
- Protein: 30g
- Fat: 26g
- Fiber: 1g
- Sugar: 4g

Number of Serves: 4
Cooking Time: 20 minutes

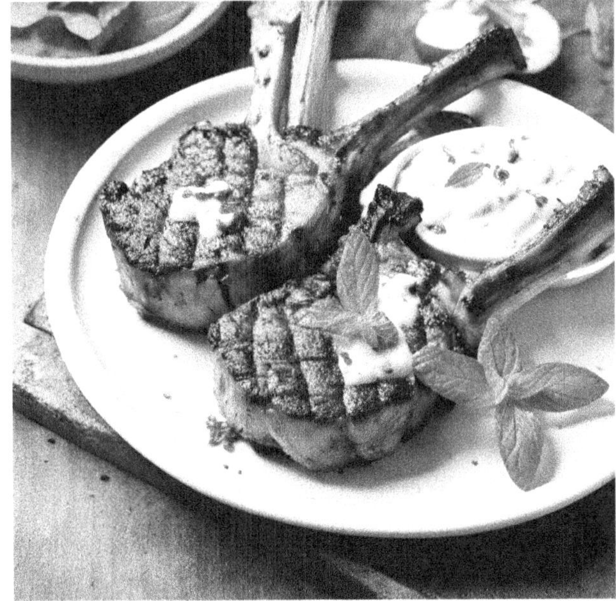

4. Lamb Tagine with Apricots

Ingredients:

- 1 1/2 lbs lamb shoulder, cut into 1-inch cubes
- 2 tablespoons olive oil
- 1 large onion, diced
- 3 cloves garlic, minced
- 1 teaspoon ground cinnamon
- 1 teaspoon ground cumin
- 1 teaspoon ground ginger
- 1/2 teaspoon ground turmeric
- 1/4 teaspoon ground black pepper
- 1/4 teaspoon sea salt
- 1/4 teaspoon saffron threads (optional)
- 2 cups chicken broth (low sodium)
- 1 cup dried apricots, halved
- 1/4 cup almonds, toasted
- Fresh cilantro, chopped (for garnish)
- Cooked couscous, for serving

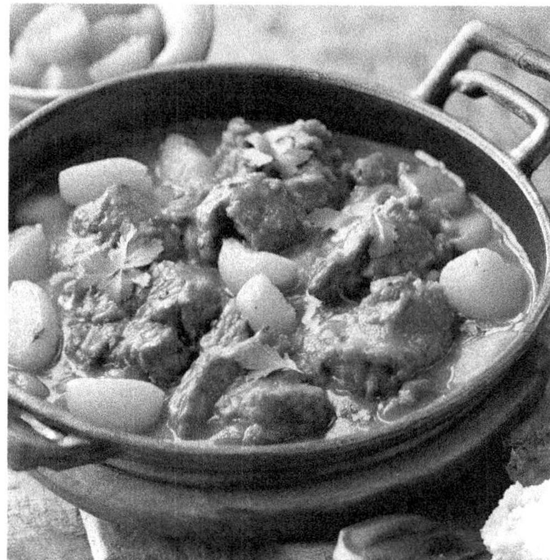

Instructions:

1. Heat the olive oil in a large pot or Dutch oven over medium-high heat.
2. Add the lamb cubes, sea salt, and black pepper, browning on all sides, about 5-7 minutes. Remove and set aside.
3. In the same pot, add the onion and garlic, sautéing for 3-4 minutes until softened.
4. Stir in the cinnamon, cumin, ginger, turmeric, and saffron threads (if using), cooking for another minute.
5. Return the lamb to the pot and add the chicken broth.
6. Bring to a boil, then reduce heat to low and simmer for 1 1/2 hours, or until the lamb is tender.
7. Add the dried apricots and continue to simmer for an additional 15 minutes.
8. Stir in the toasted almonds.
9. Serve hot over cooked couscous, garnished with fresh cilantro.

Nutrition Info (per serving):

- Calories: 450
- Carbohydrates: 40g
- Protein: 28g
- Fat: 20g
- Fiber: 6g
- Sugar: 20g

Number of Serves: 4

Cooking Time: 2 hours

5. Grilled Beef Skewers

Ingredients:

- 1 lb beef sirloin, cut into 1-inch cubes
- 2 bell peppers (any color), cut into 1-inch pieces
- 1 red onion, cut into 1-inch pieces
- 1 zucchini, sliced into rounds
- 2 tablespoons olive oil
- 2 tablespoons soy sauce (low sodium)
- 1 tablespoon lemon juice
- 2 cloves garlic, minced
- 1 teaspoon dried oregano
- 1/4 teaspoon sea salt
- 1/4 teaspoon black pepper
- Wooden skewers, soaked in water for 30 minutes

Instructions:

1. In a large bowl, mix the olive oil, soy sauce, lemon juice, garlic, oregano, sea salt, and black pepper.
2. Add the beef cubes to the marinade and toss to coat. Let marinate for at least 30 minutes.
3. Preheat the grill to medium-high heat.
4. Thread the beef, bell peppers, red onion, and zucchini onto the soaked wooden skewers.
5. Grill the skewers for 8-10 minutes, turning occasionally, until the beef is cooked to your desired doneness.
6. Serve immediately.

Nutrition Info (per serving):

- Calories: 250
- Carbohydrates: 10g
- Protein: 28g
- Fat: 12g
- Fiber: 3g
- Sugar: 5g

Number of Serves: 4

Cooking Time: 45 minutes (including marinating time)

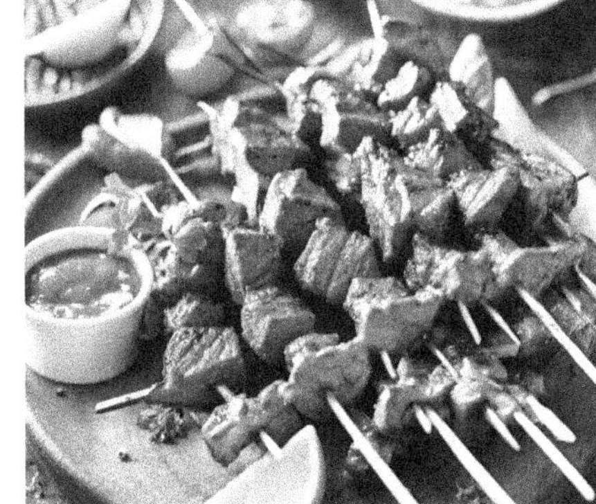

6. Beef and Barley Soup

Ingredients:

- 1 lb beef stew meat, cut into 1-inch cubes
- 2 tablespoons olive oil
- 1 large onion, diced
- 3 cloves garlic, minced
- 3 large carrots, sliced
- 3 celery stalks, sliced
- 1 cup pearl barley, rinsed
- 8 cups beef broth (low sodium)
- 1 teaspoon dried thyme
- 1 teaspoon dried rosemary
- 1 bay leaf
- 1/4 teaspoon sea salt
- 1/4 teaspoon black pepper
- 1 cup chopped kale (optional)

Instructions:

1. Heat the olive oil in a large pot over medium-high heat.
2. Add the beef, sea salt, and black pepper, browning on all sides, about 5-7 minutes. Remove and set aside.
3. In the same pot, add the onion and garlic, sautéing for 3-4 minutes until softened.
4. Add the carrots, celery, and barley, cooking for another 2-3 minutes.
5. Return the beef to the pot and add the beef broth, thyme, rosemary, and bay leaf.
6. Bring to a boil, then reduce heat to low and simmer for 1 1/2 to 2 hours, or until the beef and barley are tender.
7. Stir in the chopped kale during the last 10 minutes of cooking, if using.
8. Remove the bay leaf before serving.
9. Serve hot.

Nutrition Info (per serving):

- Calories: 320
- Carbohydrates: 35g
- Protein: 28g
- Fat: 10g
- Fiber: 6g
- Sugar: 6g

Number of Serves: 6

Cooking Time: 2 hours

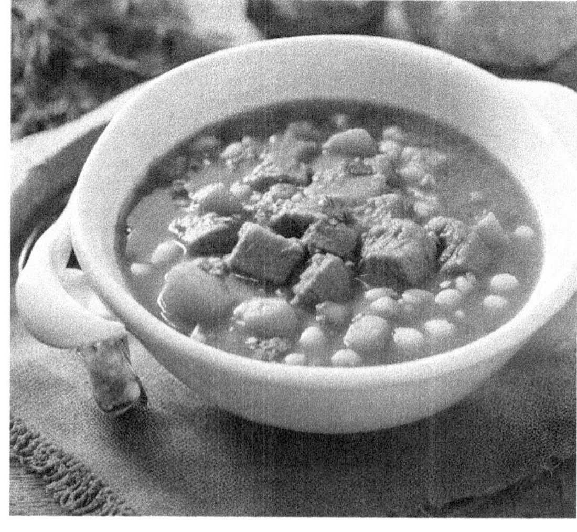

7. Slow Cooker Pot Roast

Ingredients:

- 3 lbs beef chuck roast
- 2 tablespoons olive oil
- 1 large onion, sliced
- 4 cloves garlic, minced
- 4 large carrots, peeled and cut into chunks
- 3 large potatoes, cut into chunks
- 2 cups beef broth (low sodium)
- 1 cup water
- 1 tablespoon tomato paste
- 1 teaspoon dried thyme
- 1 teaspoon dried rosemary
- 1 bay leaf
- 1/4 teaspoon sea salt
- 1/4 teaspoon black pepper

Instructions:

1. Heat the olive oil in a large skillet over medium-high heat.
2. Season the beef chuck roast with sea salt and black pepper, and brown on all sides in the skillet, about 4-5 minutes per side.
3. Transfer the roast to a slow cooker.
4. Add the onion, garlic, carrots, and potatoes to the slow cooker.
5. In a bowl, mix the beef broth, water, tomato paste, thyme, rosemary, and bay leaf.
6. Pour the mixture over the beef and vegetables.
7. Cover and cook on low for 8-10 hours, or until the beef is tender.
8. Remove the bay leaf before serving.
9. Serve hot.

Nutrition Info (per serving):

- Calories: 400
- Carbohydrates: 25g
- Protein: 30g
- Fat: 20g
- Fiber: 5g
- Sugar: 6g

Number of Serves: 6
Cooking Time: 8-10 hours

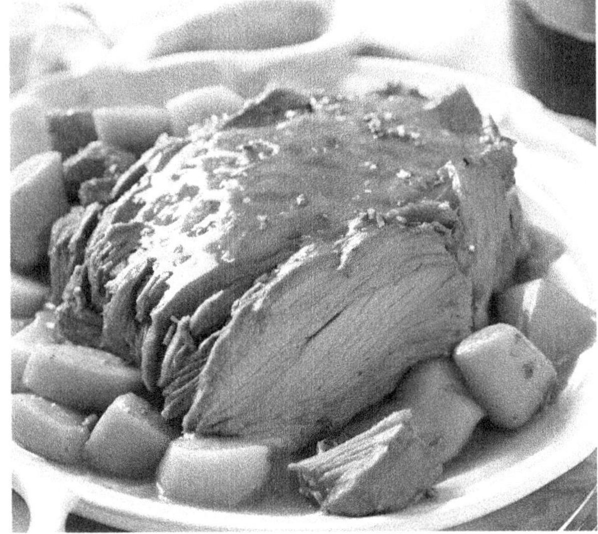

8. Spiced Beef Patties

Ingredients:

- 1 lb ground beef
- 1/4 cup finely chopped onion
- 2 cloves garlic, minced
- 1 teaspoon ground cumin
- 1 teaspoon paprika
- 1/2 teaspoon ground coriander
- 1/4 teaspoon ground cinnamon
- 1/4 teaspoon sea salt
- 1/4 teaspoon black pepper
- 1 tablespoon olive oil (for cooking)

Instructions:

1. In a large bowl, combine the ground beef, onion, garlic, cumin, paprika, coriander, cinnamon, sea salt, and black pepper. Mix until well combined.
2. Form the mixture into 8 small patties.
3. Heat the olive oil in a large skillet over medium-high heat.
4. Cook the patties for 4-5 minutes per side, or until cooked through.
5. Serve hot with your favorite sides.

Nutrition Info (per serving):

- Calories: 200
- Carbohydrates: 2g
- Protein: 20g
- Fat: 12g
- Fiber: 1g
- Sugar: 1g

Number of Serves: 4
Cooking Time: 20 minutes

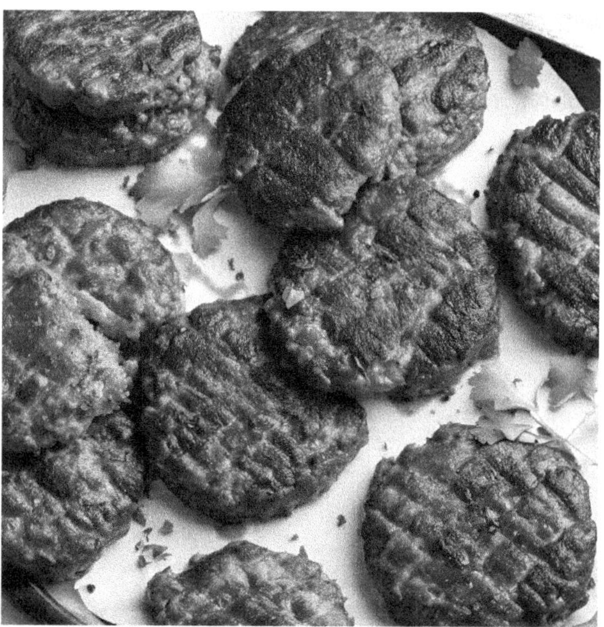

9. Beef and Spinach Lasagna

Ingredients:

- 1 lb ground beef
- 1 large onion, diced
- 3 cloves garlic, minced
- 1 (24 oz) jar marinara sauce (low sodium)
- 1 (10 oz) package frozen chopped spinach, thawed and drained
- 1 (15 oz) container ricotta cheese
- 1 large egg
- 2 cups shredded mozzarella cheese
- 1/2 cup grated Parmesan cheese
- 12 lasagna noodles (whole wheat or gluten-free), cooked
- 1 teaspoon dried basil
- 1 teaspoon dried oregano
- 1/4 teaspoon sea salt
- 1/4 teaspoon black pepper

Instructions:

1. Preheat the oven to 375°F (190°C).
2. In a large skillet, cook the ground beef, onion, and garlic over medium-high heat until the beef is browned and the onion is softened, about 7-8 minutes. Drain any excess fat.
3. Stir in the marinara sauce, basil, oregano, sea salt, and black pepper. Simmer for 10 minutes.
4. In a bowl, combine the ricotta cheese, egg, and spinach.
5. Spread a thin layer of the meat sauce in the bottom of a 9x13-inch baking dish.
6. Layer with 4 lasagna noodles, followed by 1/3 of the ricotta mixture, 1/3 of the meat sauce, and 1/3 of the mozzarella cheese. Repeat the layers twice more.
7. Sprinkle the top with Parmesan cheese.
8. Cover with foil and bake for 25 minutes. Remove the foil and bake for an additional 20 minutes, or until the cheese is melted and bubbly.
9. Let the lasagna rest for 10 minutes before serving.

Nutrition Info (per serving):

- Calories: 400
- Carbohydrates: 35g
- Protein: 30g
- Fat: 18g
- Fiber: 5g
- Sugar: 8g

Number of Serves: 8
Cooking Time: 1 hour 15 minutes

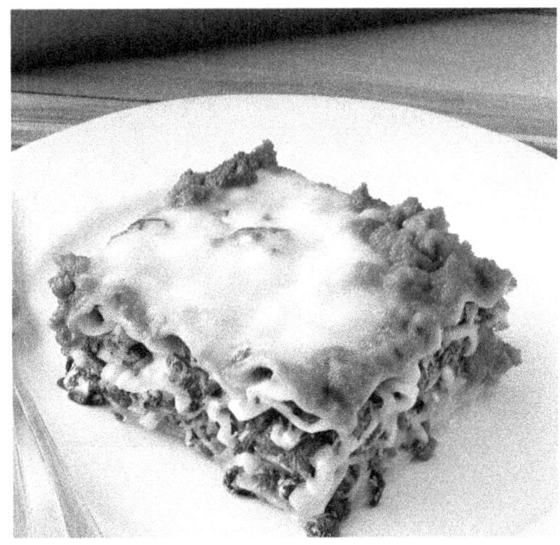

10. Balsamic Glazed Beef Roast

Ingredients:

- 3 lbs beef chuck roast
- 2 tablespoons olive oil
- 1 large onion, sliced
- 3 cloves garlic, minced
- 1/2 cup balsamic vinegar
- 1/4 cup beef broth (low sodium)
- 1/4 cup honey
- 2 tablespoons tomato paste
- 1 teaspoon dried thyme
- 1/4 teaspoon sea salt
- 1/4 teaspoon black pepper

Instructions:

1. Preheat the oven to 325°F (165°C).
2. Heat the olive oil in a large oven-safe pot or Dutch oven over medium-high heat.
3. Season the beef chuck roast with sea salt and black pepper, and brown on all sides in the pot, about 4-5 minutes per side. Remove and set aside.
4. In the same pot, add the onion and garlic, sautéing for 3-4 minutes until softened.
5. Stir in the balsamic vinegar, beef broth, honey, tomato paste, and thyme.
6. Return the beef to the pot, spooning some of the sauce over the top.
7. Cover and roast in the oven for 2 1/2 to 3 hours, or until the beef is tender.
8. Remove the beef from the pot and let rest for 10 minutes before slicing.
9. Serve with the balsamic glaze sauce.

Nutrition Info (per serving):

- Calories: 350
- Carbohydrates: 20g
- Protein: 30g
- Fat: 16g
- Fiber: 2g
- Sugar: 15g

Number of Serves: 6

Cooking Time: 3 hours

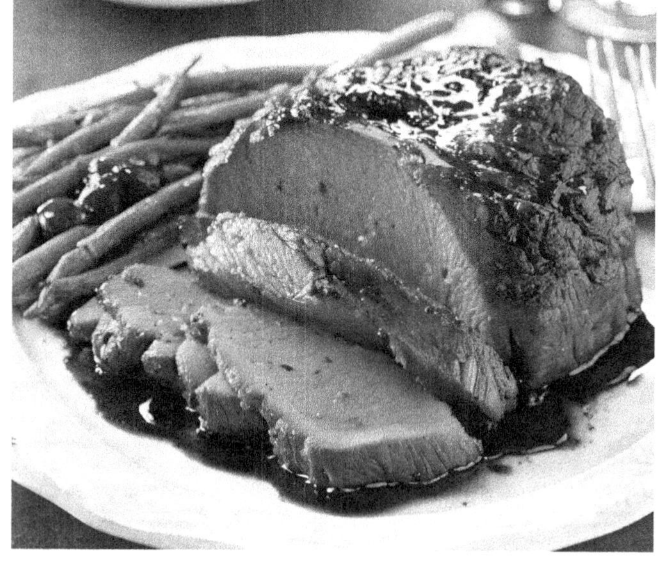

11. Beef Tenderloin with Roasted Vegetables

Ingredients:

- 2 lbs beef tenderloin
- 2 tablespoons olive oil
- 4 cloves garlic, minced
- 1 tablespoon fresh rosemary, chopped
- 1 teaspoon sea salt
- 1/2 teaspoon black pepper
- 4 large carrots, peeled and cut into chunks
- 2 large parsnips, peeled and cut into chunks
- 2 red bell peppers, sliced
- 1 large red onion, sliced
- 2 tablespoons balsamic vinegar

Instructions:

1. Preheat the oven to 400°F (200°C).
2. In a small bowl, mix the olive oil, garlic, rosemary, sea salt, and black pepper. Rub the mixture all over the beef tenderloin.
3. Place the tenderloin on a roasting rack in a large baking dish.
4. In a separate bowl, toss the carrots, parsnips, bell peppers, and onion with balsamic vinegar, sea salt, and black pepper.
5. Arrange the vegetables around the tenderloin in the baking dish.
6. Roast for 25-30 minutes for medium-rare, or until the internal temperature reaches 135°F (57°C). Adjust time for desired doneness.
7. Let the beef rest for 10 minutes before slicing.
8. Serve the tenderloin slices with the roasted vegetables.

Nutrition Info (per serving):

- Calories: 350
- Carbohydrates: 20g
- Protein: 32g
- Fat: 16g
- Fiber: 6g
- Sugar: 10g

Number of Serves: 6

Cooking Time: 40 minutes

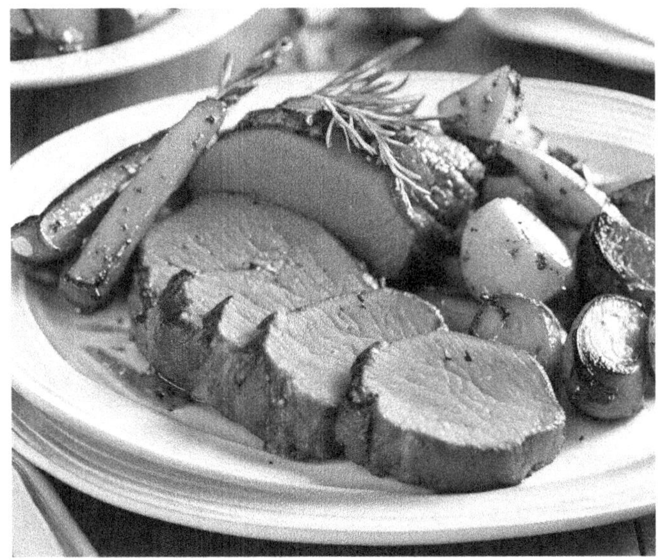

12. Korean Beef Bibimbap

Ingredients:

- 1 lb ground beef
- 2 tablespoons soy sauce (low sodium)
- 1 tablespoon sesame oil
- 2 cloves garlic, minced
- 1 tablespoon honey or maple syrup
- 1 teaspoon fresh ginger, grated
- 1 cup cooked brown rice
- 1 cup spinach, wilted
- 1 carrot, julienned
- 1 cucumber, sliced
- 4 large eggs, fried
- 2 green onions, sliced
- 1 tablespoon sesame seeds

Instructions:

1. In a skillet, cook the ground beef over medium heat until browned, about 5-7 minutes.
2. Add the soy sauce, sesame oil, garlic, honey or maple syrup, and ginger to the skillet. Cook for an additional 2-3 minutes, stirring frequently.
3. To assemble, divide the cooked brown rice among four bowls.
4. Top each bowl with the cooked beef, wilted spinach, julienned carrot, sliced cucumber, and a fried egg.
5. Sprinkle with green onions and sesame seeds.
6. Serve immediately.

Nutrition Info (per serving):

- Calories: 400
- Carbohydrates: 30g
- Protein: 25g
- Fat: 20g
- Fiber: 4g
- Sugar: 8g

Number of Serves: 4

Cooking Time: 20 minutes

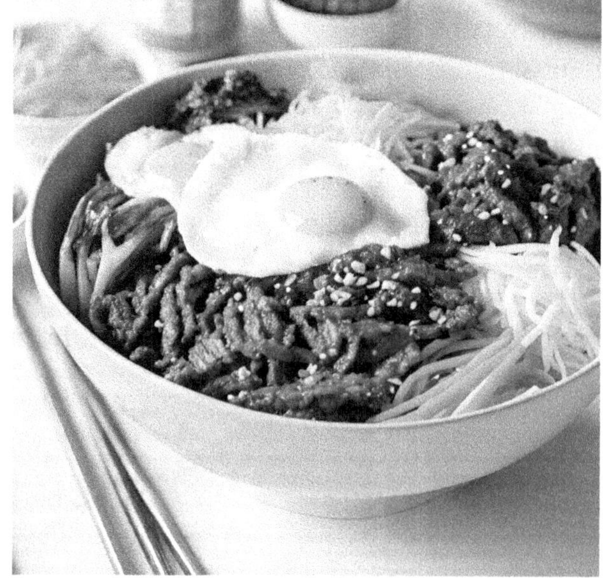

13. Meatloaf with Tomato Glaze

Ingredients:

- 1 1/2 lbs ground beef
- 1 small onion, finely chopped
- 2 cloves garlic, minced
- 1/2 cup rolled oats
- 1/2 cup almond milk (unsweetened)
- 1 large egg
- 2 tablespoons ketchup (low sugar)
- 1 tablespoon Worcestershire sauce
- 1 teaspoon dried thyme
- 1/2 teaspoon sea salt
- 1/4 teaspoon black pepper
- 1/4 cup ketchup (for glaze)
- 1 tablespoon honey or maple syrup (for glaze)

Instructions:

1. Preheat the oven to 375°F (190°C) and line a baking sheet with parchment paper.
2. In a large bowl, combine the ground beef, onion, garlic, rolled oats, almond milk, egg, 2 tablespoons ketchup, Worcestershire sauce, thyme, sea salt, and black pepper. Mix until well combined.
3. Shape the mixture into a loaf and place it on the prepared baking sheet.
4. In a small bowl, mix the 1/4 cup ketchup and honey or maple syrup for the glaze.
5. Spread the glaze evenly over the meatloaf.
6. Bake for 45-50 minutes, or until the meatloaf is cooked through and the internal temperature reaches 160°F (71°C).
7. Let the meatloaf rest for 10 minutes before slicing.
8. Serve hot.

Nutrition Info (per serving):

- Calories: 300
- Carbohydrates: 15g
- Protein: 25g
- Fat: 16g
- Fiber: 2g
- Sugar: 8g

Number of Serves: 6
Cooking Time: 1 hour

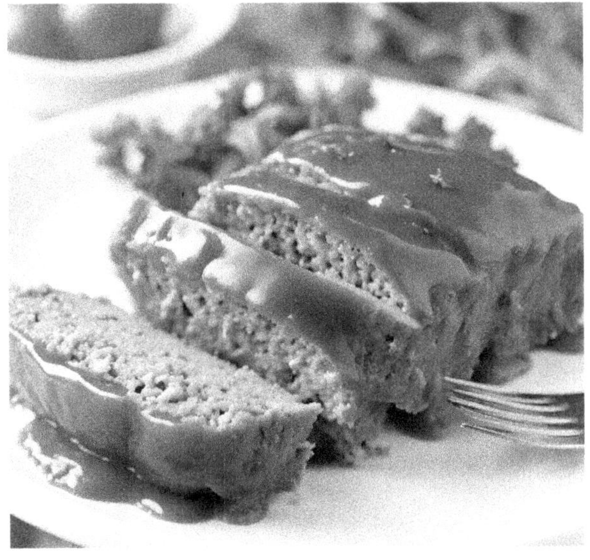

14. Beef Gyros

Ingredients:

- 1 lb beef sirloin, thinly sliced
- 2 tablespoons olive oil
- 2 cloves garlic, minced
- 1 teaspoon dried oregano
- 1 teaspoon dried thyme
- 1/2 teaspoon sea salt
- 1/4 teaspoon black pepper
- 4 whole wheat pita breads
- 1 cup Greek yogurt (unsweetened)
- 1 cucumber, finely chopped
- 1 small onion, finely chopped
- 1 tablespoon lemon juice
- Fresh dill, chopped (for garnish)
- Sliced tomatoes (for serving)
- Sliced red onions (for serving)

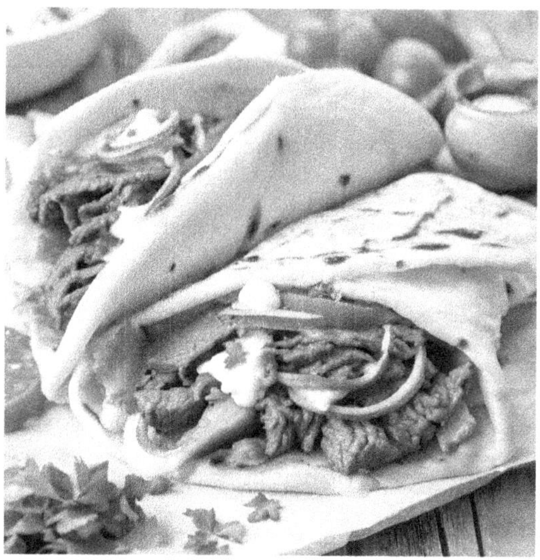

Instructions:

1. In a large bowl, combine the beef slices, olive oil, garlic, oregano, thyme, sea salt, and black pepper. Mix well and let marinate for at least 30 minutes.
2. Preheat a skillet over medium-high heat.
3. Cook the beef in the skillet until browned and cooked through, about 5-7 minutes.
4. In a small bowl, mix the Greek yogurt, cucumber, onion, and lemon juice to make the tzatziki sauce.
5. Warm the pita breads in the oven or on a skillet.
6. Assemble the gyros by placing the cooked beef on the pita breads, topping with tzatziki sauce, sliced tomatoes, and sliced red onions.
7. Garnish with fresh dill and serve immediately.

Nutrition Info (per serving):

- Calories: 350
- Carbohydrates: 30g
- Protein: 25g
- Fat: 14g
- Fiber: 4g
- Sugar: 6g

Number of Serves: 4

Cooking Time: 40 minutes (including marinating time)

15. Beef Pho

Ingredients:

- 1 lb beef sirloin, thinly sliced
- 8 cups beef broth (low sodium)
- 4 cups water
- 1 onion, halved
- 4 cloves garlic, smashed
- 3-inch piece ginger, sliced
- 2 star anise
- 4 cloves
- 1 cinnamon stick
- 1 tablespoon fish sauce
- 1 tablespoon soy sauce (low sodium)
- 1 lb rice noodles
- Fresh basil, for garnish
- Fresh cilantro, for garnish
- Sliced jalapeños, for garnish
- Bean sprouts, for garnish
- Lime wedges, for serving

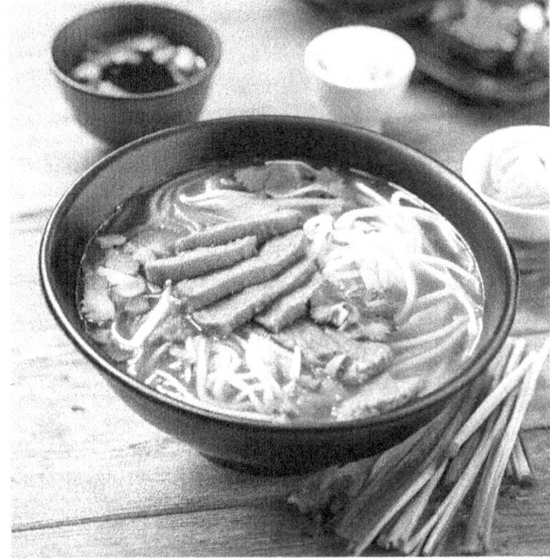

Instructions:

1. In a large pot, combine the beef broth, water, onion, garlic, ginger, star anise, cloves, and cinnamon stick. Bring to a boil, then reduce heat and simmer for 30 minutes.
2. Strain the broth to remove the solids, then return the broth to the pot.
3. Stir in the fish sauce and soy sauce.
4. Cook the rice noodles according to package instructions, then drain and set aside.
5. To serve, divide the cooked rice noodles among bowls.
6. Top with the thinly sliced beef sirloin.
7. Ladle the hot broth over the beef and noodles, allowing the heat of the broth to cook the beef.
8. Garnish with fresh basil, cilantro, sliced jalapeños, and bean sprouts.
9. Serve with lime wedges.

Nutrition Info (per serving):

- Calories: 350
- Carbohydrates: 45g
- Protein: 25g
- Fat: 8g
- Fiber: 3g
- Sugar: 4g

Number of Serves: 4

Cooking Time: 45 minutes

16. Sloppy Joes

Ingredients:

- 1 lb ground beef
- 1 small onion, diced
- 1 green bell pepper, diced
- 2 cloves garlic, minced
- 1 (15 oz) can tomato sauce (low sodium)
- 1/4 cup ketchup (low sugar)
- 2 tablespoons Worcestershire sauce
- 1 tablespoon brown sugar
- 1 teaspoon dried mustard
- 1/4 teaspoon sea salt
- 1/4 teaspoon black pepper
- 4 whole wheat hamburger buns

Instructions:

1. In a large skillet, cook the ground beef over medium-high heat until browned, about 5-7 minutes. Drain any excess fat.
2. Add the onion, bell pepper, and garlic to the skillet, cooking until softened, about 3-4 minutes.
3. Stir in the tomato sauce, ketchup, Worcestershire sauce, brown sugar, dried mustard, sea salt, and black pepper.
4. Simmer for 10-15 minutes, stirring occasionally, until the mixture thickens.
5. Toast the whole wheat hamburger buns.
6. Serve the sloppy joe mixture on the toasted buns.

Nutrition Info (per serving):

- Calories: 320
- Carbohydrates: 35g
- Protein: 20g
- Fat: 12g
- Fiber: 5g
- Sugar: 12g

Number of Serves: 4
Cooking Time: 30 minutes

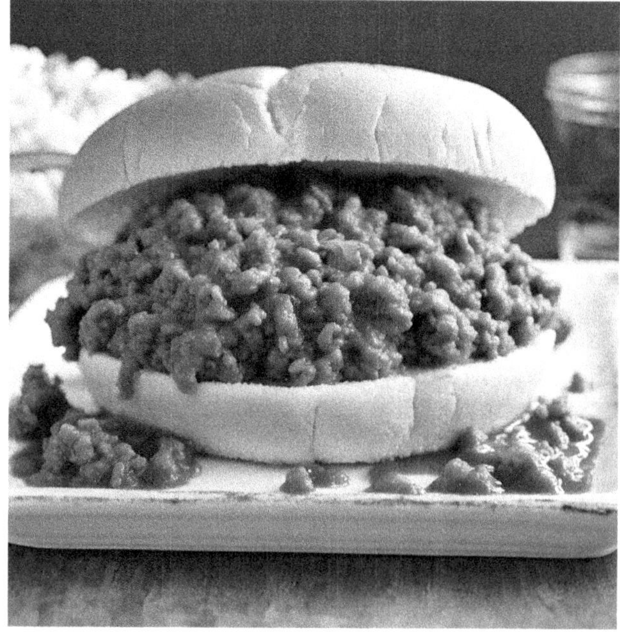

17. Beef and Mushroom Stroganoff

Ingredients:

- 1 lb beef sirloin, thinly sliced
- 2 tablespoons olive oil
- 1 large onion, diced
- 3 cloves garlic, minced
- 8 oz mushrooms, sliced
- 2 tablespoons all-purpose flour
- 1 cup beef broth (low sodium)
- 1 cup almond milk (unsweetened)
- 1 tablespoon Dijon mustard
- 1/2 teaspoon sea salt
- 1/4 teaspoon black pepper
- 1/2 cup Greek yogurt (unsweetened)
- Cooked whole wheat egg noodles, for serving
- Fresh parsley, chopped (for garnish)

Instructions:

1. Heat the olive oil in a large skillet over medium-high heat.
2. Add the sliced beef, sea salt, and black pepper, browning on all sides, about 4-5 minutes. Remove and set aside.
3. In the same skillet, add the onion and garlic, sautéing for 3-4 minutes until softened.
4. Add the mushrooms and cook for another 5 minutes until they release their moisture and begin to brown.
5. Stir in the flour and cook for 1-2 minutes.
6. Gradually add the beef broth and almond milk, stirring constantly until the mixture thickens.
7. Stir in the Dijon mustard.
8. Return the beef to the skillet and simmer for 5-7 minutes until heated through.
9. Remove from heat and stir in the Greek yogurt.
10. Serve the stroganoff over cooked whole wheat egg noodles, garnished with fresh parsley.

Nutrition Info (per serving):

- Calories: 350
- Carbohydrates: 30g
- Protein: 28g
- Fat: 12g
- Fiber: 4g
- Sugar: 6g

Number of Serves: 4
Cooking Time: 30 minutes

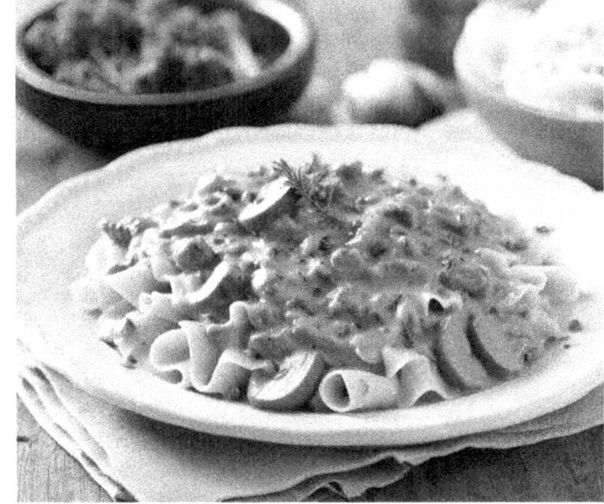

18. Roast Lamb with Rosemary and Garlic

Ingredients:

- 4 lbs leg of lamb
- 4 cloves garlic, sliced
- 2 tablespoons fresh rosemary, chopped
- 2 tablespoons olive oil
- 1 teaspoon sea salt
- 1/2 teaspoon black pepper
- 1 lemon, cut into wedges (for serving)

Instructions:

1. Preheat the oven to 375°F (190°C).
2. Using a sharp knife, make small slits all over the leg of lamb and insert the garlic slices into the slits.
3. Rub the lamb with olive oil, rosemary, sea salt, and black pepper.
4. Place the lamb in a roasting pan and roast for 1 1/2 to 2 hours, or until the internal temperature reaches 145°F (63°C) for medium-rare.
5. Let the lamb rest for 10 minutes before carving.
6. Serve with lemon wedges.

Nutrition Info (per serving):

- Calories: 400
- Carbohydrates: 2g
- Protein: 30g
- Fat: 30g
- Fiber: 0g
- Sugar: 0g

Number of Serves: 8

Cooking Time: 2 hours

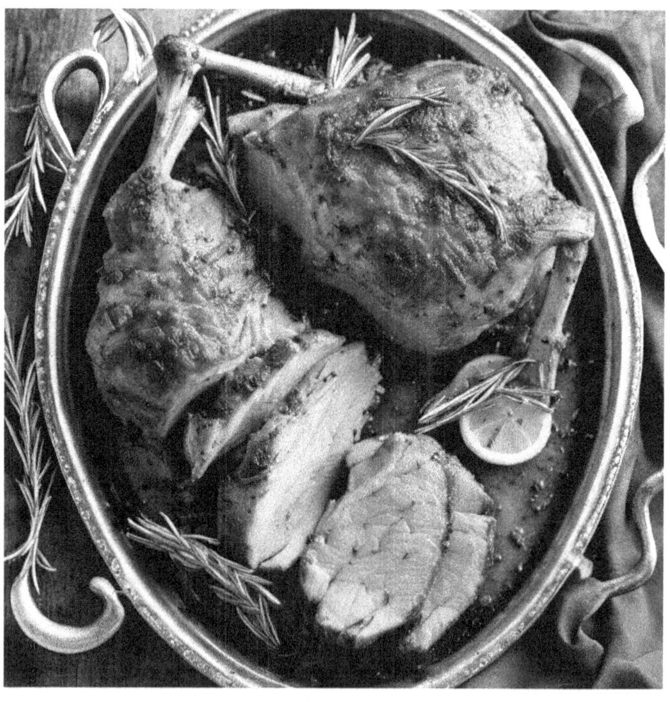

19. Lamb Curry with Coconut Milk

Ingredients:

- 1 1/2 lbs lamb shoulder, cut into 1-inch cubes
- 2 tablespoons olive oil
- 1 large onion, diced
- 3 cloves garlic, minced
- 1 tablespoon ginger, minced
- 2 tablespoons curry powder
- 1 teaspoon ground cumin
- 1 teaspoon ground coriander
- 1/2 teaspoon turmeric
- 1/2 teaspoon sea salt
- 1/4 teaspoon black pepper
- 1 (14 oz) can coconut milk
- 1 cup chicken broth (low sodium)
- 1 cup diced tomatoes
- 1 cup baby spinach
- Fresh cilantro, chopped (for garnish)
- Cooked brown rice, for serving

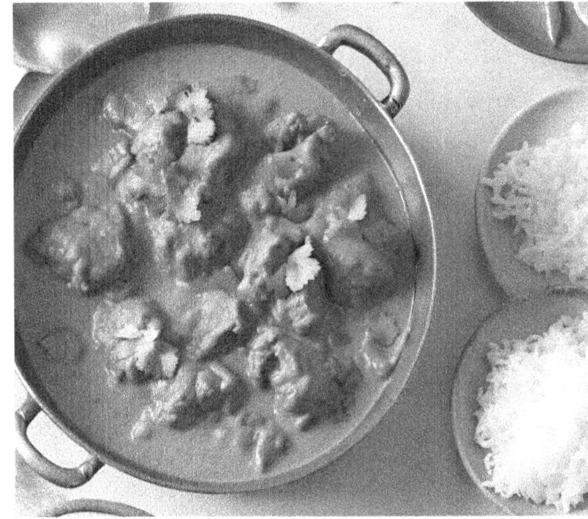

Instructions:

1. Heat the olive oil in a large pot over medium-high heat.
2. Add the lamb and brown on all sides, about 5-7 minutes. Remove and set aside.
3. In the same pot, add the onion, garlic, and ginger. Sauté for 3-4 minutes until softened.
4. Stir in the curry powder, cumin, coriander, turmeric, sea salt, and black pepper. Cook for another minute until fragrant.
5. Add the coconut milk, chicken broth, and diced tomatoes. Bring to a boil.
6. Return the lamb to the pot, reduce heat to low, and simmer for 1 1/2 hours, or until the lamb is tender.
7. Stir in the baby spinach and cook for an additional 5 minutes.
8. Serve hot over cooked brown rice, garnished with fresh cilantro.

Nutrition Info (per serving):

- Calories: 450
- Carbohydrates: 25g
- Protein: 28g
- Fat: 26g
- Fiber: 4g
- Sugar: 6g

Number of Serves: 6

Cooking Time: 2 hours

20. Lamb and Lentil Stew

Ingredients:

- 1 1/2 lbs lamb shoulder, cut into 1-inch cubes
- 2 tablespoons olive oil
- 1 large onion, diced
- 3 cloves garlic, minced
- 2 large carrots, sliced
- 3 celery stalks, sliced
- 1 cup dried green lentils, rinsed
- 6 cups chicken broth (low sodium)
- 1 teaspoon dried thyme
- 1 teaspoon dried rosemary
- 1/2 teaspoon sea salt
- 1/4 teaspoon black pepper
- 2 cups baby spinach
- Fresh parsley, chopped (for garnish)

Instructions:

1. Heat the olive oil in a large pot over medium-high heat.
2. Add the lamb and brown on all sides, about 5-7 minutes. Remove and set aside.
3. In the same pot, add the onion, garlic, carrots, and celery. Sauté for 5-7 minutes until softened.
4. Stir in the lentils, chicken broth, thyme, rosemary, sea salt, and black pepper.
5. Bring to a boil, then reduce heat to low and simmer for 1 1/2 hours, or until the lentils and lamb are tender.
6. Stir in the baby spinach and cook for an additional 5 minutes.
7. Serve hot, garnished with fresh parsley.

Nutrition Info (per serving):

- Calories: 350
- Carbohydrates: 35g
- Protein: 28g
- Fat: 12g
- Fiber: 10g
- Sugar: 6g

Number of Serves: 6

Cooking Time: 2 hours

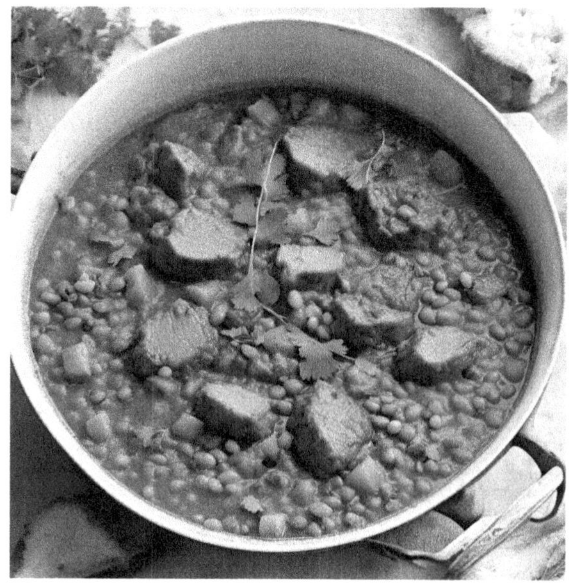

21. Mediterranean Lamb Meatballs

Ingredients:

- 1 lb ground lamb
- 1/4 cup finely chopped onion
- 2 cloves garlic, minced
- 1/4 cup chopped fresh parsley
- 1 teaspoon ground cumin
- 1 teaspoon ground coriander
- 1/2 teaspoon ground cinnamon
- 1/2 teaspoon sea salt
- 1/4 teaspoon black pepper
- 2 tablespoons olive oil (for cooking)
- 1 cup Greek yogurt (unsweetened)
- 1 cucumber, finely chopped
- 1 tablespoon lemon juice
- Fresh mint, chopped (for garnish)

Instructions:

1. In a large bowl, combine the ground lamb, onion, garlic, parsley, cumin, coriander, cinnamon, sea salt, and black pepper. Mix until well combined.
2. Form the mixture into small meatballs.
3. Heat the olive oil in a large skillet over medium-high heat.
4. Cook the meatballs for 5-7 minutes per side, or until cooked through.
5. In a small bowl, mix the Greek yogurt, cucumber, and lemon juice to make the tzatziki sauce.
6. Serve the meatballs with the tzatziki sauce, garnished with fresh mint.

Nutrition Info (per serving):

- Calories: 300
- Carbohydrates: 10g
- Protein: 20g
- Fat: 20g
- Fiber: 1g
- Sugar: 4g

Number of Serves: 4
Cooking Time: 25 minutes

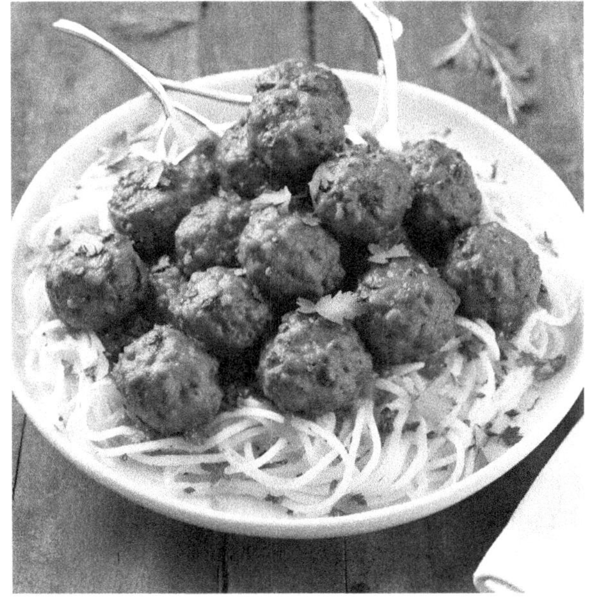

22. Lamb Shank Braised in Red Wine

Ingredients:

- 4 lamb shanks
- 2 tablespoons olive oil
- 1 large onion, diced
- 3 cloves garlic, minced
- 2 carrots, peeled and sliced
- 2 celery stalks, sliced
- 2 cups red wine
- 2 cups beef broth (low sodium)
- 1 (14 oz) can diced tomatoes
- 1 tablespoon tomato paste
- 1 teaspoon dried rosemary
- 1 teaspoon dried thyme
- 1 bay leaf
- 1/2 teaspoon sea salt
- 1/4 teaspoon black pepper

Instructions:

1. Preheat the oven to 325°F (165°C).
2. Heat the olive oil in a large oven-safe pot or Dutch oven over medium-high heat.
3. Season the lamb shanks with sea salt and black pepper, and brown on all sides, about 5-7 minutes. Remove and set aside.
4. In the same pot, add the onion, garlic, carrots, and celery. Sauté for 5-7 minutes until softened.
5. Stir in the red wine, beef broth, diced tomatoes, tomato paste, rosemary, thyme, and bay leaf. Bring to a boil.
6. Return the lamb shanks to the pot, spooning some of the sauce over the top.
7. Cover and transfer to the oven. Braise for 2 1/2 to 3 hours, or until the lamb is tender.
8. Remove the bay leaf before serving.
9. Serve hot.

Nutrition Info (per serving):

- Calories: 450
- Carbohydrates: 15g
- Protein: 35g
- Fat: 25g
- Fiber: 4g
- Sugar: 6g

Number of Serves: 4

Cooking Time: 3 hours

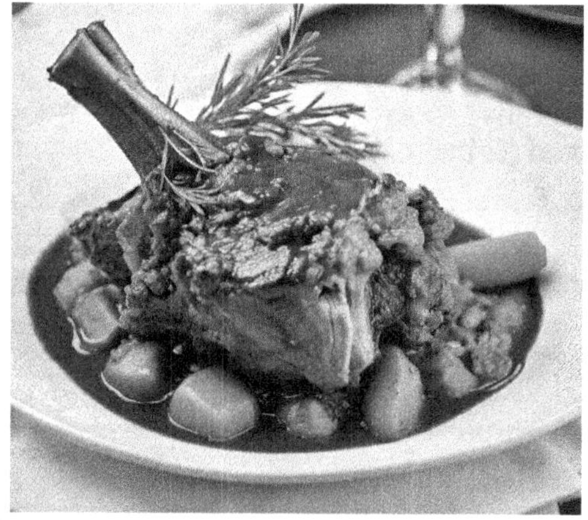

23. Lamb Gyros with Greek Salad

Ingredients:

- 1 lb ground lamb
- 2 cloves garlic, minced
- 1 teaspoon dried oregano
- 1 teaspoon ground cumin
- 1/2 teaspoon sea salt
- 1/4 teaspoon black pepper
- 4 whole wheat pita breads
- 1 cup Greek yogurt (unsweetened)
- 1 cucumber, finely chopped
- 1 small onion, finely chopped
- 1 tablespoon lemon juice
- Fresh dill, chopped (for garnish)
- Sliced tomatoes (for serving)
- Sliced red onions (for serving)

Instructions:

1. In a large bowl, combine the ground lamb, garlic, oregano, cumin, sea salt, and black pepper. Mix well and form into patties.
2. Preheat a skillet over medium-high heat.
3. Cook the lamb patties for 5-7 minutes per side, or until cooked through.
4. In a small bowl, mix the Greek yogurt, cucumber, onion, and lemon juice to make the tzatziki sauce.
5. Warm the pita breads in the oven or on a skillet.
6. Assemble the gyros by placing the cooked lamb patties on the pita breads, topping with tzatziki sauce, sliced tomatoes, and sliced red onions.
7. Garnish with fresh dill and serve immediately.

Nutrition Info (per serving):

- Calories: 350
- Carbohydrates: 30g
- Protein: 25g
- Fat: 14g
- Fiber: 4g
- Sugar: 6g

Number of Serves: 4
Cooking Time: 30 minutes

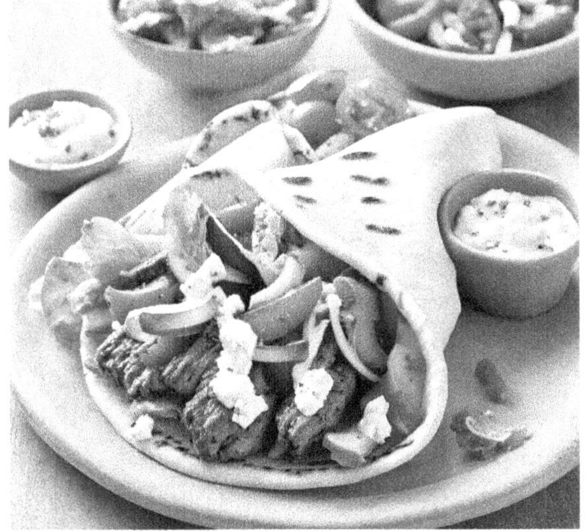

24. Lamb Biryani

Ingredients:

- 1 1/2 lbs lamb shoulder, cut into 1-inch cubes
- 2 cups basmati rice
- 4 cups water
- 2 tablespoons olive oil
- 1 large onion, sliced
- 3 cloves garlic, minced
- 1 tablespoon ginger, minced
- 1 cup Greek yogurt (unsweetened)
- 1 teaspoon ground turmeric
- 1 teaspoon ground cumin
- 1 teaspoon ground coriander
- 1 teaspoon garam masala
- 1/2 teaspoon sea salt
- 1/4 teaspoon black pepper
- 1/4 cup fresh mint, chopped
- 1/4 cup fresh cilantro, chopped
- 1/2 cup slivered almonds (optional)
- Saffron threads (optional, soaked in 2 tablespoons warm milk)

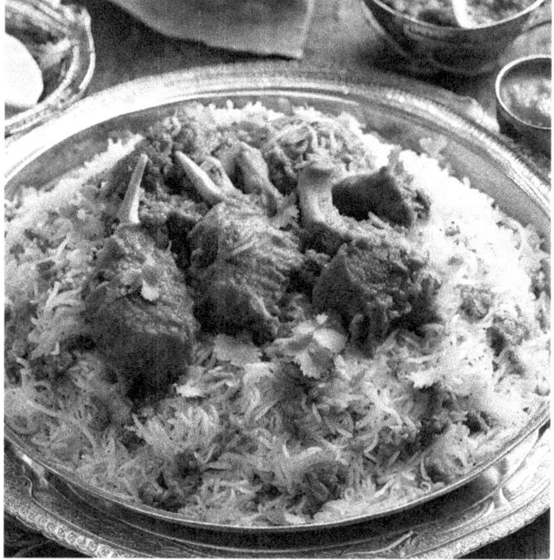

Instructions:

1. Rinse the basmati rice under cold water until the water runs clear. Soak in water for 30 minutes, then drain.
2. Heat the olive oil in a large pot over medium-high heat.
3. Add the lamb and brown on all sides, about 5-7 minutes. Remove and set aside.
4. In the same pot, add the onion, garlic, and ginger. Sauté for 3-4 minutes until softened.
5. Stir in the turmeric, cumin, coriander, garam masala, sea salt, and black pepper.
6. Return the lamb to the pot and stir in the Greek yogurt. Cook for 5 minutes, stirring occasionally.
7. Add the basmati rice and water to the pot. Bring to a boil, then reduce heat to low.
8. Cover and cook for 20-25 minutes, or until the rice is tender and the liquid is absorbed.
9. Stir in the fresh mint, cilantro, and slivered almonds (if using). Drizzle with saffron milk if using.
10. Serve hot.

Nutrition Info (per serving):

- Calories: 450 Carbohydrates: 55g Protein: 25g Fat: 16g Fiber: 4g
- Sugar: 6g

Number of Serves: 6

Cooking Time: 1 hour

25. Lamb Koftas with Tzatziki

Ingredients:

- 1 lb ground lamb
- 1/4 cup finely chopped onion
- 2 cloves garlic, minced
- 1/4 cup fresh parsley, chopped
- 1 teaspoon ground cumin
- 1 teaspoon ground coriander
- 1/2 teaspoon ground cinnamon
- 1/2 teaspoon sea salt
- 1/4 teaspoon black pepper
- 2 tablespoons olive oil (for cooking)
- 1 cup Greek yogurt (unsweetened)
- 1 cucumber, finely chopped
- 1 tablespoon lemon juice
- Fresh mint, chopped (for garnish)

Instructions:

1. In a large bowl, combine the ground lamb, onion, garlic, parsley, cumin, coriander, cinnamon, sea salt, and black pepper. Mix until well combined.
2. Form the mixture into small sausage-shaped koftas.
3. Heat the olive oil in a large skillet over medium-high heat.
4. Cook the koftas for 5-7 minutes per side, or until cooked through.
5. In a small bowl, mix the Greek yogurt, cucumber, and lemon juice to make the tzatziki sauce.
6. Serve the koftas with the tzatziki sauce, garnished with fresh mint.

Nutrition Info (per serving):

- Calories: 300
- Carbohydrates: 10g
- Protein: 20g
- Fat: 20g
- Fiber: 1g
- Sugar: 4g

Number of Serves: 4
Cooking Time: 25 minutes

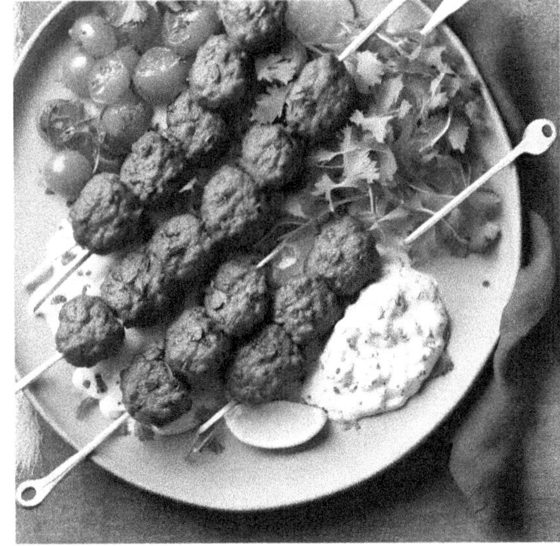

26. Shepherd's Pie with Sweet Potato Topping

Ingredients:

- 1 1/2 lbs ground lamb
- 1 large onion, diced
- 3 cloves garlic, minced
- 2 large carrots, diced
- 2 celery stalks, diced
- 1 cup frozen peas
- 1 cup beef broth (low sodium)
- 2 tablespoons tomato paste
- 1 teaspoon dried thyme
- 1 teaspoon dried rosemary
- 1/2 teaspoon sea salt
- 1/4 teaspoon black pepper
- 4 large sweet potatoes, peeled and cubed
- 1/4 cup almond milk (unsweetened)
- 2 tablespoons olive oil

Instructions:

1. Preheat the oven to 375°F (190°C).
2. In a large pot, boil the sweet potatoes until tender, about 15 minutes. Drain and mash with almond milk and olive oil. Set aside.
3. In a large skillet, cook the ground lamb over medium-high heat until browned, about 5-7 minutes. Drain any excess fat.
4. Add the onion, garlic, carrots, and celery to the skillet. Sauté for 5-7 minutes until softened.
5. Stir in the tomato paste, beef broth, thyme, rosemary, sea salt, and black pepper. Cook for an additional 5 minutes.
6. Add the frozen peas and cook for another 2 minutes.
7. Transfer the lamb mixture to a baking dish and spread the mashed sweet potatoes evenly on top.
8. Bake for 20-25 minutes, or until the top is slightly golden.
9. Serve hot.

Nutrition Info (per serving):

- Calories: 400
- Carbohydrates: 45g
- Protein: 25g
- Fat: 16g
- Fiber: 8g
- Sugar: 12g

Number of Serves: 6

Cooking Time: 1 hour

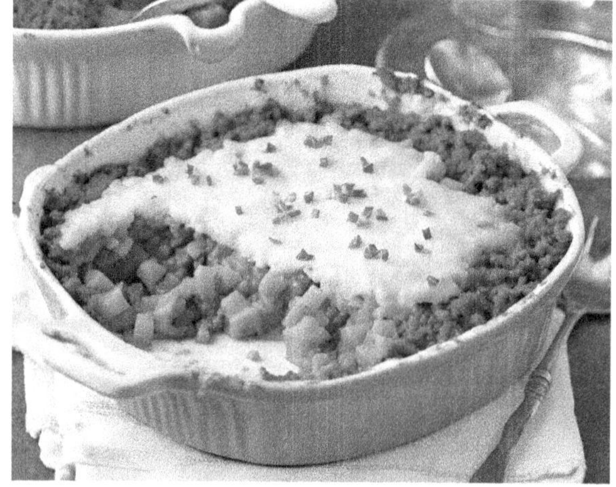

27. Lamb Stuffed Eggplants

Ingredients:

- 4 small eggplants, halved and flesh scooped out
- 1 lb ground lamb
- 1 small onion, diced
- 2 cloves garlic, minced
- 1 cup diced tomatoes
- 1/2 cup cooked quinoa
- 1 teaspoon ground cumin
- 1 teaspoon ground coriander
- 1/2 teaspoon sea salt
- 1/4 teaspoon black pepper
- 1/4 cup fresh parsley, chopped
- 1/4 cup grated Parmesan cheese (optional)

Instructions:

1. Preheat the oven to 375°F (190°C).
2. Place the eggplant halves on a baking sheet and roast for 20 minutes, or until tender.
3. In a large skillet, cook the ground lamb, onion, and garlic over medium-high heat until the lamb is browned and the onion is softened, about 7-8 minutes.
4. Stir in the diced tomatoes, cooked quinoa, cumin, coriander, sea salt, and black pepper. Cook for another 5 minutes.
5. Remove the eggplants from the oven and fill them with the lamb mixture.
6. Sprinkle with grated Parmesan cheese if desired.
7. Return to the oven and bake for an additional 10-15 minutes.
8. Garnish with fresh parsley and serve hot.

Nutrition Info (per serving):

- Calories: 350
- Carbohydrates: 20g
- Protein: 25g
- Fat: 18g
- Fiber: 6g
- Sugar: 8g

Number of Serves: 4
Cooking Time: 45 minutes

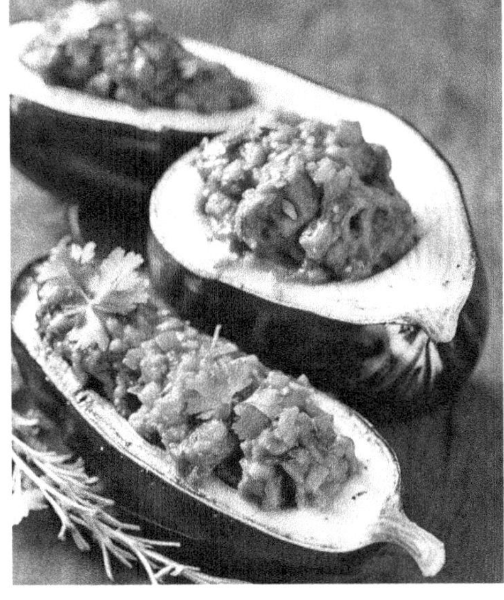

28. Irish Lamb Stew

Ingredients:

- 2 lbs lamb shoulder, cut into 1-inch cubes
- 2 tablespoons olive oil
- 1 large onion, diced
- 3 cloves garlic, minced
- 4 large carrots, sliced
- 4 large potatoes, peeled and diced
- 4 cups beef broth (low sodium)
- 1 cup water
- 1 teaspoon dried thyme
- 1 teaspoon dried rosemary
- 1 bay leaf
- 1/2 teaspoon sea salt
- 1/4 teaspoon black pepper
- Fresh parsley, chopped (for garnish)

Instructions:

1. Heat the olive oil in a large pot over medium-high heat.
2. Add the lamb and brown on all sides, about 5-7 minutes. Remove and set aside.
3. In the same pot, add the onion and garlic. Sauté for 3-4 minutes until softened.
4. Stir in the carrots, potatoes, beef broth, water, thyme, rosemary, bay leaf, sea salt, and black pepper.
5. Return the lamb to the pot and bring to a boil.
6. Reduce heat to low and simmer for 1 1/2 to 2 hours, or until the lamb and vegetables are tender.
7. Remove the bay leaf before serving.
8. Garnish with fresh parsley and serve hot.

Nutrition Info (per serving):

- Calories: 400
- Carbohydrates: 30g
- Protein: 28g
- Fat: 18g
- Fiber: 6g
- Sugar: 6g

Number of Serves: 6

Cooking Time: 2 hours

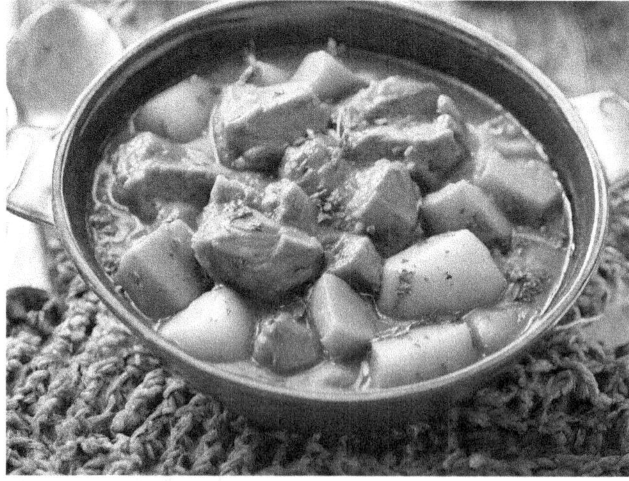

29. Rack of Lamb with Herb Crust

Ingredients:

- 2 racks of lamb (about 8 ribs each)
- 2 tablespoons olive oil
- 4 cloves garlic, minced
- 2 tablespoons fresh rosemary, chopped
- 2 tablespoons fresh thyme, chopped
- 1/2 cup bread crumbs (whole wheat)
- 1/4 cup grated Parmesan cheese (optional)
- 1 teaspoon sea salt
- 1/2 teaspoon black pepper

Instructions:

1. Preheat the oven to 425°F (220°C).
2. In a small bowl, mix the olive oil, garlic, rosemary, thyme, bread crumbs, Parmesan cheese (if using), sea salt, and black pepper.
3. Rub the mixture all over the lamb racks.
4. Place the lamb on a baking sheet and roast for 25-30 minutes, or until the internal temperature reaches 145°F (63°C) for medium-rare.
5. Let the lamb rest for 10 minutes before slicing.
6. Serve hot.

Nutrition Info (per serving):

- Calories: 450
- Carbohydrates: 10g
- Protein: 30g
- Fat: 32g
- Fiber: 2g
- Sugar: 1g

Number of Serves: 4
Cooking Time: 40 minutes

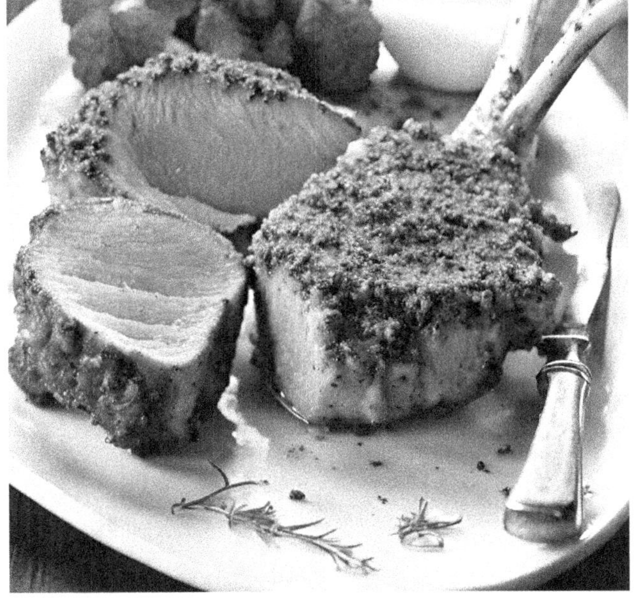

30. Lamb Skewers with Saffron Rice

Ingredients:

- 1 1/2 lbs lamb shoulder, cut into 1-inch cubes
- 2 tablespoons olive oil
- 2 cloves garlic, minced
- 1 tablespoon fresh rosemary, chopped
- 1 teaspoon ground cumin
- 1/2 teaspoon sea salt
- 1/4 teaspoon black pepper
- Wooden skewers, soaked in water for 30 minutes
- 2 cups basmati rice
- 4 cups water
- 1/2 teaspoon saffron threads, soaked in 2 tablespoons warm water
- 1 tablespoon butter
- Fresh parsley, chopped (for garnish)

Instructions:

1. In a large bowl, mix the olive oil, garlic, rosemary, cumin, sea salt, and black pepper. Add the lamb cubes and toss to coat. Let marinate for at least 30 minutes.
2. Thread the marinated lamb onto the soaked wooden skewers.
3. Preheat the grill to medium-high heat.
4. Grill the lamb skewers for 8-10 minutes, turning occasionally, until the lamb is cooked to your desired doneness.
5. Meanwhile, rinse the basmati rice under cold water until the water runs clear.
6. In a large pot, bring the water to a boil. Add the rinsed rice and saffron water, then reduce heat to low.
7. Cover and cook for 15-20 minutes, or until the rice is tender and the liquid is absorbed.
8. Stir in the butter and fluff the rice with a fork.
9. Serve the lamb skewers over the saffron rice, garnished with fresh parsley.

Nutrition Info (per serving):

- Calories: 500
- Carbohydrates: 55g
- Protein: 28g
- Fat: 20g
- Fiber: 4g
- Sugar: 2g

Number of Serves: 6

Cooking Time: 45 minutes

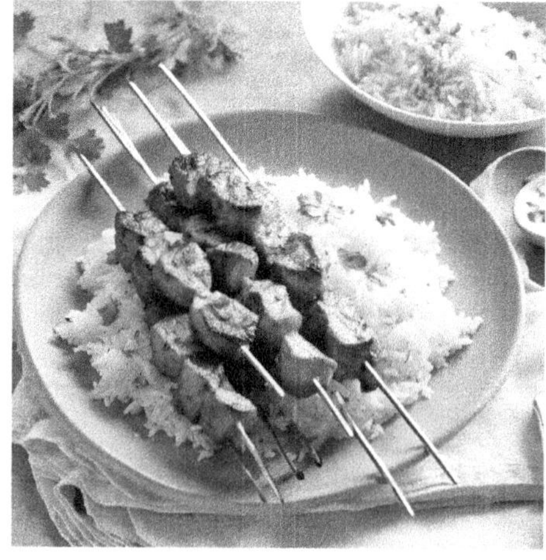

Fish and Seafood Recipes

1. Grilled Salmon with Lemon and Herbs

Ingredients:

- 4 salmon fillets (about 6 oz each)
- 2 tablespoons olive oil
- 2 cloves garlic, minced
- 1 lemon, sliced
- 2 tablespoons fresh dill, chopped
- 2 tablespoons fresh parsley, chopped
- 1/2 teaspoon sea salt
- 1/4 teaspoon black pepper

Instructions:

1. Preheat the grill to medium-high heat.
2. In a small bowl, mix the olive oil, garlic, dill, parsley, sea salt, and black pepper.
3. Rub the mixture evenly over the salmon fillets.
4. Place the lemon slices on the grill, then place the salmon fillets on top of the lemon slices.
5. Grill the salmon for 4-5 minutes per side, or until the fish flakes easily with a fork.
6. Serve hot, garnished with additional fresh herbs if desired.

Nutrition Info (per serving):

- Calories: 350
- Carbohydrates: 2g
- Protein: 34g
- Fat: 22g
- Fiber: 0g
- Sugar: 0g

Number of Serves: 4

Cooking Time: 15 minutes

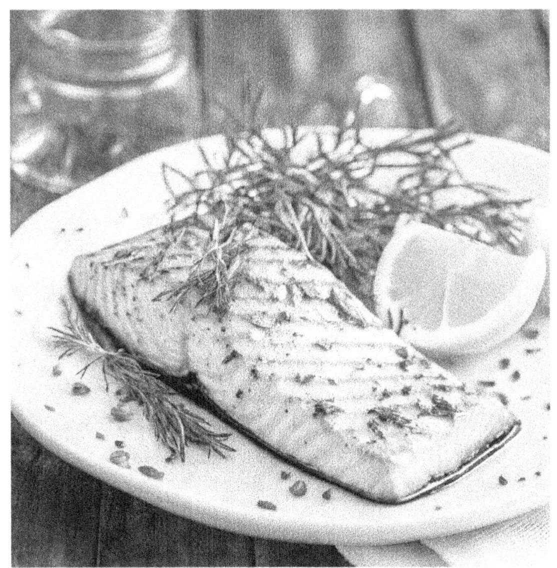

2. Baked Cod with Olive Tapenade

Ingredients:
- 4 cod fillets (about 6 oz each)
- 2 tablespoons olive oil
- 1 cup pitted Kalamata olives
- 2 cloves garlic, minced
- 1 tablespoon capers
- 2 tablespoons fresh parsley, chopped
- 1 tablespoon lemon juice
- 1/2 teaspoon sea salt
- 1/4 teaspoon black pepper

Instructions:
1. Preheat the oven to 400°F (200°C).
2. In a food processor, combine the olives, garlic, capers, parsley, lemon juice, sea salt, and black pepper. Pulse until finely chopped.
3. Place the cod fillets on a baking sheet lined with parchment paper.
4. Spread the olive tapenade evenly over the cod fillets.
5. Drizzle with olive oil.
6. Bake for 15-20 minutes, or until the fish flakes easily with a fork.
7. Serve hot.

Nutrition Info (per serving):
- Calories: 250
- Carbohydrates: 2g
- Protein: 34g
- Fat: 12g
- Fiber: 1g
- Sugar: 0g

Number of Serves: 4
Cooking Time: 25 minutes

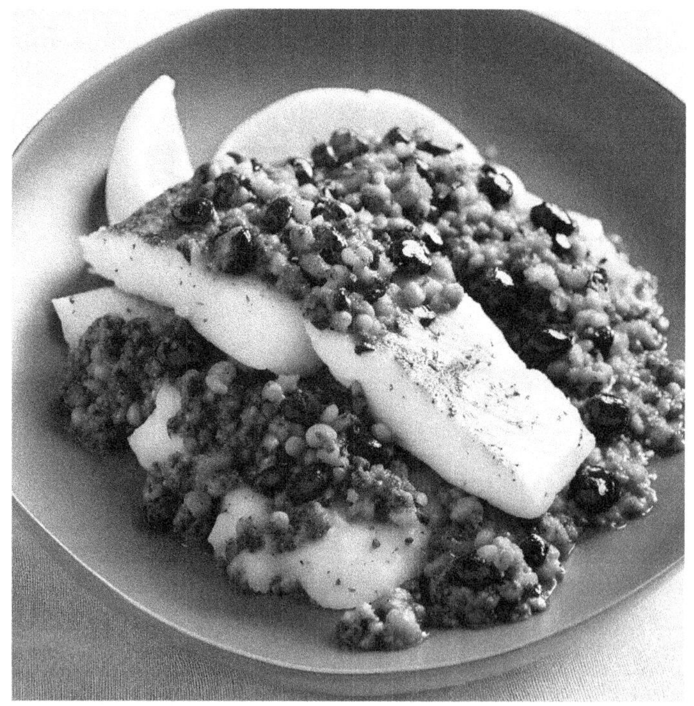

3. Pan-Seared Tilapia with Lime Butter Sauce

Ingredients:

- 4 tilapia fillets (about 6 oz each)
- 2 tablespoons olive oil
- 1/4 teaspoon sea salt
- 1/4 teaspoon black pepper
- 1/4 cup unsalted butter
- 2 cloves garlic, minced
- Juice of 2 limes
- 2 tablespoons fresh cilantro, chopped

Instructions:

1. Season the tilapia fillets with sea salt and black pepper.
2. Heat the olive oil in a large skillet over medium-high heat.
3. Add the tilapia fillets and cook for 3-4 minutes per side, or until the fish is golden brown and flakes easily with a fork. Remove from the skillet and set aside.
4. In the same skillet, melt the butter over medium heat.
5. Add the garlic and cook for 1 minute, until fragrant.
6. Stir in the lime juice and cook for another 1-2 minutes, until the sauce has slightly thickened.
7. Return the tilapia to the skillet and spoon the lime butter sauce over the fillets.
8. Garnish with fresh cilantro and serve hot.

Nutrition Info (per serving):

- Calories: 320
- Carbohydrates: 2g
- Protein: 34g
- Fat: 20g
- Fiber: 0g
- Sugar: 0g

Number of Serves: 4
Cooking Time: 15 minutes

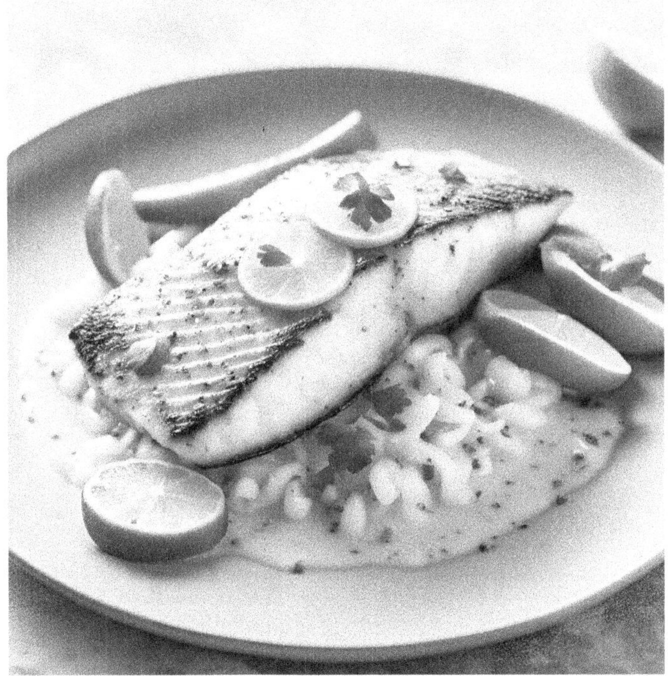

4. Spicy Tuna Poke Bowl

Ingredients:

- 1 lb sushi-grade tuna, diced
- 2 tablespoons soy sauce (low sodium)
- 1 tablespoon sesame oil
- 1 tablespoon rice vinegar
- 1 teaspoon sriracha sauce
- 1 avocado, diced
- 1 cup cooked brown rice
- 1/2 cup edamame, shelled
- 1/2 cup cucumber, diced
- 2 green onions, sliced
- 1 tablespoon sesame seeds
- 1/4 cup pickled ginger (optional)

Instructions:

1. In a large bowl, combine the diced tuna, soy sauce, sesame oil, rice vinegar, and sriracha sauce. Mix well and let marinate for 10 minutes.
2. Divide the cooked brown rice among four bowls.
3. Top each bowl with the marinated tuna, avocado, edamame, cucumber, and green onions.
4. Sprinkle with sesame seeds and add pickled ginger if desired.
5. Serve immediately.

Nutrition Info (per serving):

- Calories: 400
- Carbohydrates: 30g
- Protein: 30g
- Fat: 20g
- Fiber: 6g
- Sugar: 2g

Number of Serves: 4

Cooking Time: 20 minutes

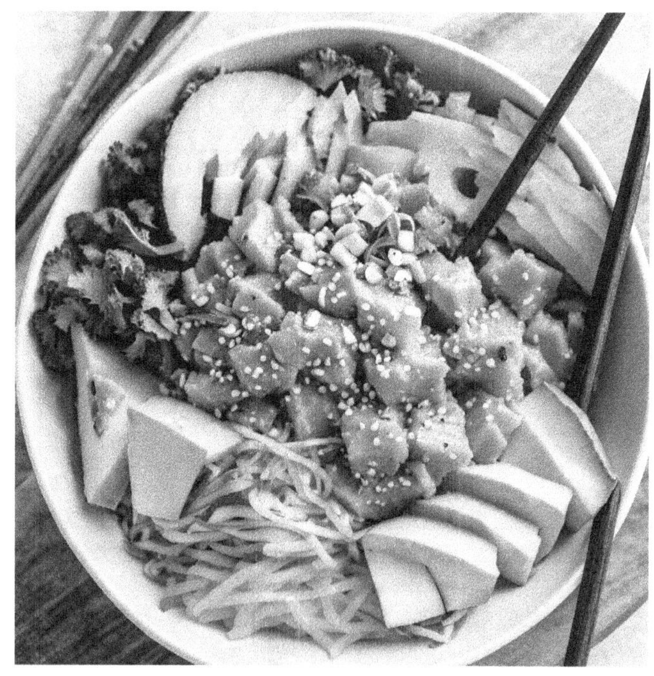

5. Herb-Crusted Haddock

Ingredients:

- 4 haddock fillets (about 6 oz each)
- 1 cup whole wheat bread crumbs
- 2 tablespoons fresh parsley, chopped
- 2 tablespoons fresh dill, chopped
- 2 cloves garlic, minced
- 1 lemon, zested
- 2 tablespoons olive oil
- 1/2 teaspoon sea salt
- 1/4 teaspoon black pepper

Instructions:

1. Preheat the oven to 400°F (200°C) and line a baking sheet with parchment paper.
2. In a bowl, combine the bread crumbs, parsley, dill, garlic, lemon zest, sea salt, and black pepper.
3. Brush the haddock fillets with olive oil and press the breadcrumb mixture onto each fillet to coat.
4. Place the fillets on the prepared baking sheet.
5. Bake for 15-20 minutes, or until the fish flakes easily with a fork and the crust is golden brown.
6. Serve hot with lemon wedges.

Nutrition Info (per serving):

- Calories: 300
- Carbohydrates: 15g
- Protein: 34g
- Fat: 12g
- Fiber: 2g
- Sugar: 1g

Number of Serves: 4
Cooking Time: 25 minutes

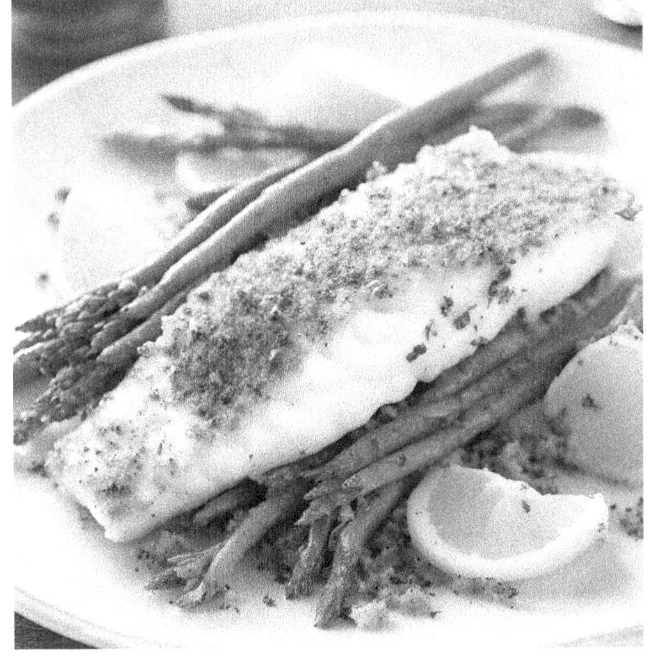

6. Sardines on Toast

Ingredients:

- 2 cans sardines in olive oil (about 4 oz each)
- 4 slices whole grain bread, toasted
- 1 small red onion, thinly sliced
- 1 lemon, juiced
- 2 tablespoons fresh parsley, chopped
- 1/4 teaspoon sea salt
- 1/4 teaspoon black pepper

Instructions:

1. Drain the sardines and place them in a bowl. Flake the sardines with a fork.
2. Add the red onion, lemon juice, parsley, sea salt, and black pepper to the bowl and mix well.
3. Toast the whole grain bread slices.
4. Top each toast slice with the sardine mixture.
5. Serve immediately.

Nutrition Info (per serving):

- Calories: 250
- Carbohydrates: 20g
- Protein: 16g
- Fat: 12g
- Fiber: 4g
- Sugar: 2g

Number of Serves: 4
Cooking Time: 10 minutes

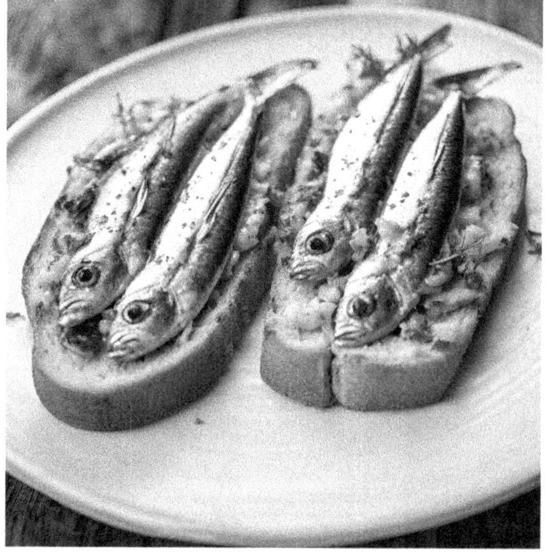

7. Salmon and Asparagus in Foil

Ingredients:

- 4 salmon fillets (about 6 oz each)
- 1 lb asparagus, trimmed
- 2 cloves garlic, minced
- 2 tablespoons olive oil
- 1 lemon, sliced
- 2 tablespoons fresh dill, chopped
- 1/2 teaspoon sea salt
- 1/4 teaspoon black pepper

Instructions:

1. Preheat the oven to 375°F (190°C).
2. Cut four large pieces of aluminum foil. Place a salmon fillet in the center of each piece.
3. Divide the asparagus evenly among the four pieces of foil, placing them next to the salmon.
4. In a small bowl, mix the garlic, olive oil, dill, sea salt, and black pepper.
5. Drizzle the olive oil mixture over the salmon and asparagus.
6. Top each fillet with lemon slices.
7. Fold the sides of the foil over the salmon and asparagus, sealing the packets.
8. Place the foil packets on a baking sheet and bake for 20-25 minutes, or until the salmon is cooked through and the asparagus is tender.
9. Serve hot.

Nutrition Info (per serving):

- Calories: 350
- Carbohydrates: 6g
- Protein: 34g
- Fat: 20g
- Fiber: 3g
- Sugar: 2g

Number of Serves: 4
Cooking Time: 30 minutes

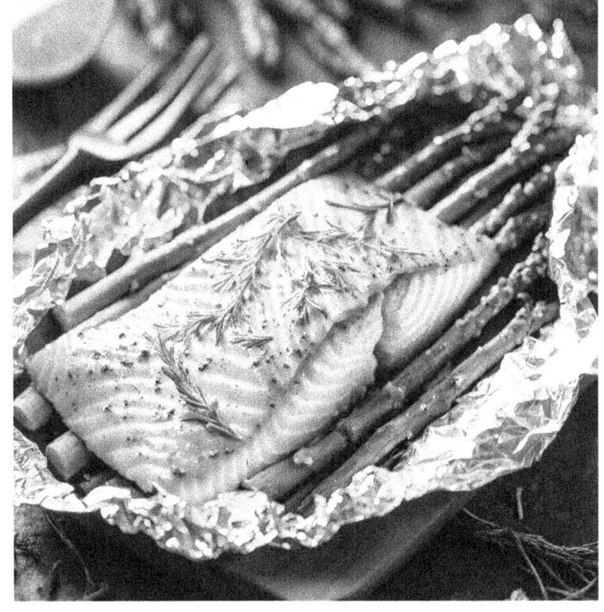

8. Fish Curry with Coconut Milk

Ingredients:

- 1 1/2 lbs white fish fillets (such as cod or tilapia), cut into chunks
- 2 tablespoons olive oil
- 1 large onion, diced
- 3 cloves garlic, minced
- 1 tablespoon ginger, minced
- 1 tablespoon curry powder
- 1 teaspoon ground turmeric
- 1 teaspoon ground cumin
- 1/2 teaspoon sea salt
- 1/4 teaspoon black pepper
- 1 (14 oz) can coconut milk
- 1 cup diced tomatoes
- 1 cup vegetable broth (low sodium)
- Fresh cilantro, chopped (for garnish)
- Cooked brown rice, for serving

Instructions:

1. Heat the olive oil in a large pot over medium heat.
2. Add the onion, garlic, and ginger, sautéing for 3-4 minutes until softened.
3. Stir in the curry powder, turmeric, cumin, sea salt, and black pepper. Cook for another minute until fragrant.
4. Add the coconut milk, diced tomatoes, and vegetable broth. Bring to a simmer.
5. Add the fish chunks and cook for 10-12 minutes, or until the fish is cooked through and flakes easily with a fork.
6. Serve the fish curry hot over cooked brown rice, garnished with fresh cilantro.

Nutrition Info (per serving):

- Calories: 400
- Carbohydrates: 20g
- Protein: 32g
- Fat: 22g
- Fiber: 4g
- Sugar: 6g

Number of Serves: 4

Cooking Time: 25 minutes

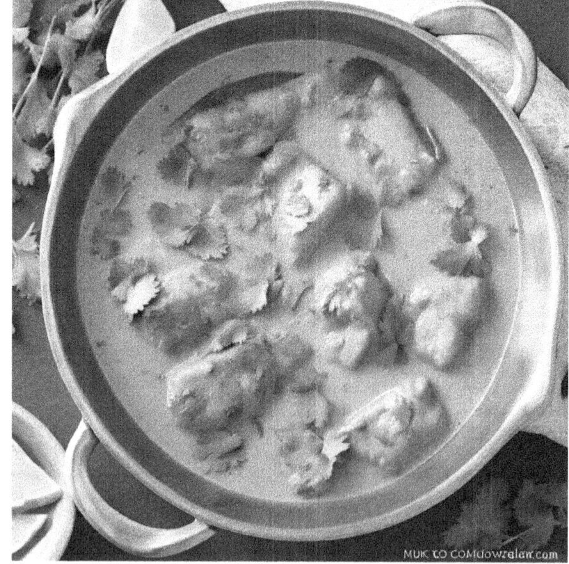

9. Trout Almondine

Ingredients:

- 4 trout fillets (about 6 oz each)
- 1/2 cup almond flour
- 1/4 teaspoon sea salt
- 1/4 teaspoon black pepper
- 2 tablespoons olive oil
- 1/4 cup unsalted butter
- 1/4 cup sliced almonds
- 2 tablespoons lemon juice
- 2 tablespoons fresh parsley, chopped

Instructions:

1. Season the trout fillets with sea salt and black pepper.
2. Dredge the fillets in almond flour, shaking off any excess.
3. Heat the olive oil in a large skillet over medium-high heat.
4. Add the trout fillets to the skillet and cook for 3-4 minutes per side, or until golden brown and cooked through. Remove from the skillet and set aside.
5. In the same skillet, melt the butter over medium heat.
6. Add the sliced almonds and cook for 2-3 minutes, or until they are golden brown.
7. Stir in the lemon juice and parsley.
8. Pour the almond butter sauce over the trout fillets.
9. Serve hot.

Nutrition Info (per serving):

- Calories: 350
- Carbohydrates: 6g
- Protein: 32g
- Fat: 22g
- Fiber: 2g
- Sugar: 1g

Number of Serves: 4
Cooking Time: 20 minutes

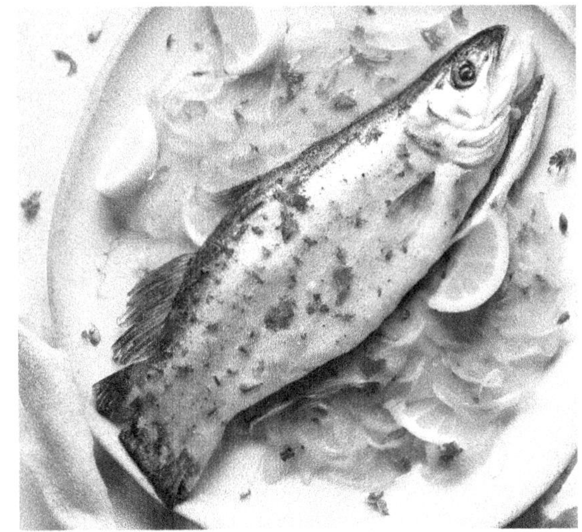

10. Mackerel Patties

Ingredients:

- 2 cans mackerel (about 15 oz each), drained and flaked
- 1/2 cup whole wheat bread crumbs
- 1 small onion, finely chopped
- 2 cloves garlic, minced
- 1 large egg, beaten
- 2 tablespoons fresh parsley, chopped
- 1 tablespoon lemon juice
- 1/4 teaspoon sea salt
- 1/4 teaspoon black pepper
- 2 tablespoons olive oil (for cooking)

Instructions:

1. In a large bowl, combine the mackerel, bread crumbs, onion, garlic, egg, parsley, lemon juice, sea salt, and black pepper. Mix until well combined.
2. Form the mixture into 8 patties.
3. Heat the olive oil in a large skillet over medium-high heat.
4. Cook the patties for 4-5 minutes per side, or until golden brown and cooked through.
5. Serve hot with lemon wedges.

Nutrition Info (per serving):

- Calories: 250
- Carbohydrates: 12g
- Protein: 24g
- Fat: 12g
- Fiber: 2g
- Sugar: 1g

Number of Serves: 4

Cooking Time: 15 minutes

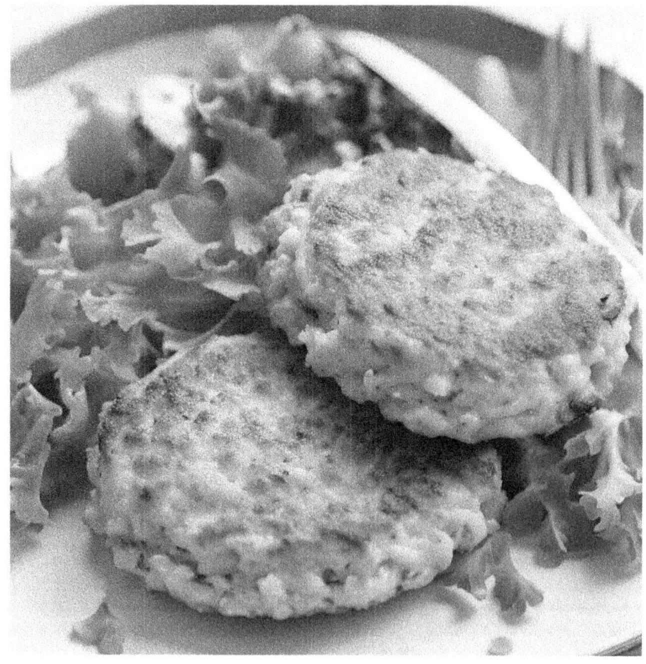

11. Sea Bass with Mediterranean Salsa

Ingredients:

- 4 sea bass fillets (about 6 oz each)
- 2 tablespoons olive oil
- 1 lemon, sliced
- 1 cup cherry tomatoes, quartered
- 1/2 cup cucumber, diced
- 1/4 cup red onion, finely chopped
- 1/4 cup Kalamata olives, pitted and sliced
- 2 tablespoons fresh parsley, chopped
- 1 tablespoon capers, drained
- 2 tablespoons lemon juice
- 1/2 teaspoon sea salt
- 1/4 teaspoon black pepper

Instructions:

1. Preheat the oven to 400°F (200°C).
2. Rub the sea bass fillets with olive oil, sea salt, and black pepper. Place them on a baking sheet lined with parchment paper.
3. Arrange the lemon slices over the fillets.
4. Bake for 15-20 minutes, or until the fish flakes easily with a fork.
5. Meanwhile, in a bowl, combine the cherry tomatoes, cucumber, red onion, olives, parsley, capers, and lemon juice.
6. Serve the baked sea bass topped with Mediterranean salsa.

Nutrition Info (per serving):

- Calories: 350
- Carbohydrates: 8g
- Protein: 34g
- Fat: 20g
- Fiber: 2g
- Sugar: 3g

Number of Serves: 4
Cooking Time: 25 minutes

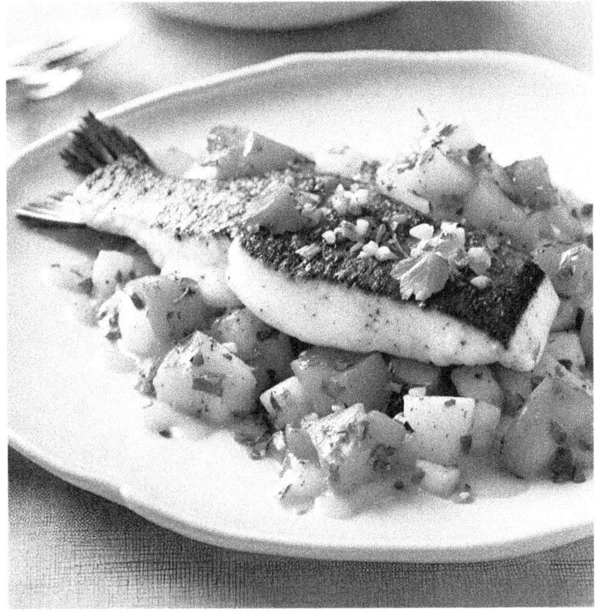

12. Catfish Étouffée

Ingredients:
- 4 catfish fillets (about 6 oz each)
- 2 tablespoons olive oil
- 1 large onion, diced
- 1 green bell pepper, diced
- 2 celery stalks, diced
- 3 cloves garlic, minced
- 1 (14 oz) can diced tomatoes
- 1 cup low sodium chicken broth
- 1 tablespoon Cajun seasoning
- 1 teaspoon smoked paprika
- 1/2 teaspoon sea salt
- 1/4 teaspoon black pepper
- 1/4 cup fresh parsley, chopped
- Cooked brown rice, for serving

Instructions:
1. Heat the olive oil in a large skillet over medium-high heat.
2. Add the onion, bell pepper, and celery. Sauté for 5-7 minutes until softened.
3. Add the garlic and cook for another minute.
4. Stir in the diced tomatoes, chicken broth, Cajun seasoning, smoked paprika, sea salt, and black pepper. Bring to a simmer.
5. Add the catfish fillets to the skillet and spoon some sauce over the top.
6. Cover and simmer for 10-12 minutes, or until the fish is cooked through and flakes easily with a fork.
7. Serve hot over cooked brown rice, garnished with fresh parsley.

Nutrition Info (per serving):
- Calories: 400
- Carbohydrates: 30g
- Protein: 34g
- Fat: 14g
- Fiber: 4g
- Sugar: 6g

Number of Serves: 4
Cooking Time: 25 minutes

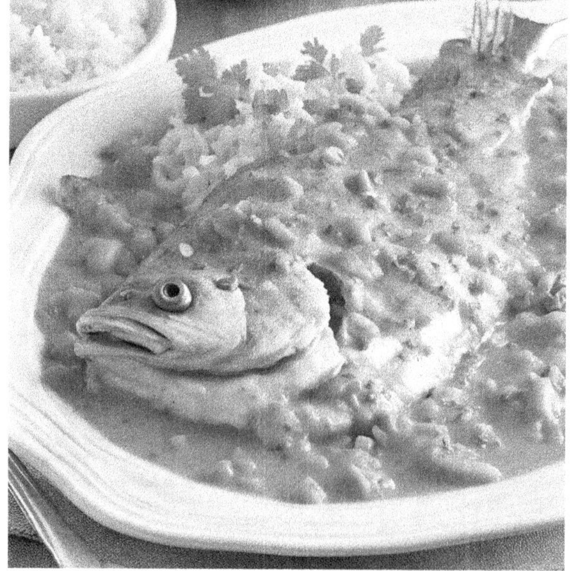

13. Baked Lemon Sole with Parmesan

Ingredients:

- 4 sole fillets (about 6 oz each)
- 2 tablespoons olive oil
- 1/2 cup grated Parmesan cheese
- 1/2 cup whole wheat bread crumbs
- 2 cloves garlic, minced
- 1 lemon, zested and juiced
- 2 tablespoons fresh parsley, chopped
- 1/2 teaspoon sea salt
- 1/4 teaspoon black pepper

Instructions:

1. Preheat the oven to 375°F (190°C) and line a baking sheet with parchment paper.
2. In a bowl, combine the Parmesan cheese, bread crumbs, garlic, lemon zest, parsley, sea salt, and black pepper.
3. Brush the sole fillets with olive oil and coat them with the Parmesan mixture.
4. Place the fillets on the prepared baking sheet.
5. Drizzle with lemon juice.
6. Bake for 15-20 minutes, or until the fish is golden brown and flakes easily with a fork.
7. Serve hot.

Nutrition Info (per serving):

- Calories: 350
- Carbohydrates: 12g
- Protein: 34g
- Fat: 18g
- Fiber: 2g
- Sugar: 1g

Number of Serves: 4
Cooking Time: 20 minutes

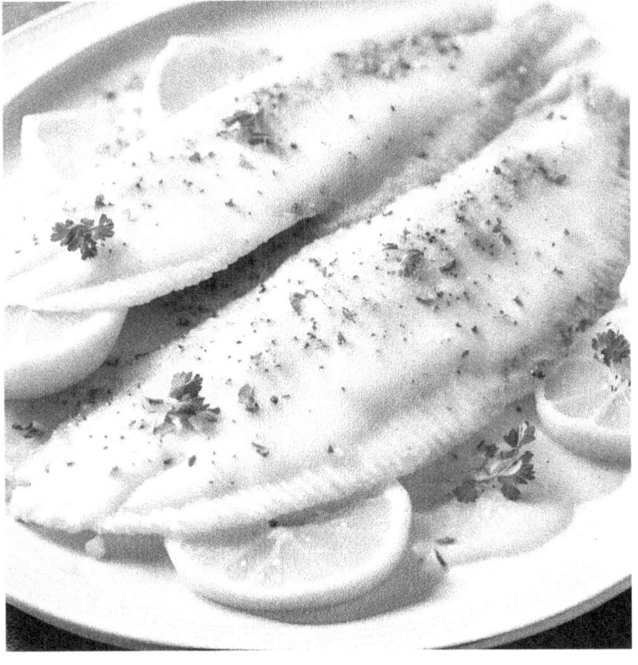

14. Anchovy Pasta with Garlic and Olive Oil

Ingredients:

- 12 oz whole wheat spaghetti
- 2 tablespoons olive oil
- 6 anchovy fillets, finely chopped
- 4 cloves garlic, minced
- 1/4 teaspoon red pepper flakes (optional)
- 1/4 cup fresh parsley, chopped
- 1 lemon, zested and juiced
- 1/2 teaspoon sea salt
- 1/4 teaspoon black pepper

Instructions:

1. Cook the spaghetti according to package instructions. Drain and set aside.
2. In a large skillet, heat the olive oil over medium heat.
3. Add the anchovy fillets and cook for 2-3 minutes until they dissolve.
4. Add the garlic and red pepper flakes (if using), cooking for another minute until fragrant.
5. Add the cooked spaghetti to the skillet and toss to coat.
6. Stir in the parsley, lemon zest, lemon juice, sea salt, and black pepper.
7. Serve hot.

Nutrition Info (per serving):

- Calories: 350
- Carbohydrates: 50g
- Protein: 14g
- Fat: 12g
- Fiber: 8g
- Sugar: 2g

Number of Serves: 4
Cooking Time: 20 minutes

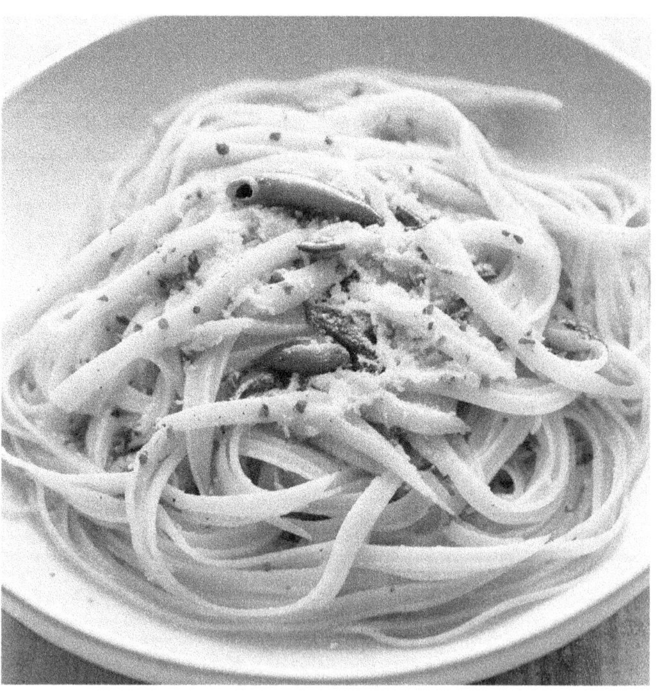

15. Halibut Steak with Caper Vinaigrette

Ingredients:

- 4 halibut steaks (about 6 oz each)
- 2 tablespoons olive oil
- 1/4 teaspoon sea salt
- 1/4 teaspoon black pepper
- 1/4 cup olive oil
- 2 tablespoons capers, rinsed and chopped
- 2 tablespoons lemon juice
- 1 tablespoon Dijon mustard
- 1 tablespoon fresh parsley, chopped
- 1 clove garlic, minced

Instructions:

1. Preheat the grill to medium-high heat.
2. Brush the halibut steaks with 2 tablespoons of olive oil and season with sea salt and black pepper.
3. Grill the halibut steaks for 4-5 minutes per side, or until the fish is cooked through and flakes easily with a fork.
4. Meanwhile, in a small bowl, whisk together 1/4 cup olive oil, capers, lemon juice, Dijon mustard, parsley, and garlic.
5. Serve the grilled halibut steaks drizzled with caper vinaigrette.

Nutrition Info (per serving):

- Calories: 400
- Carbohydrates: 2g
- Protein: 34g
- Fat: 28g
- Fiber: 1g
- Sugar: 0g

Number of Serves: 4
Cooking Time: 15 minutes

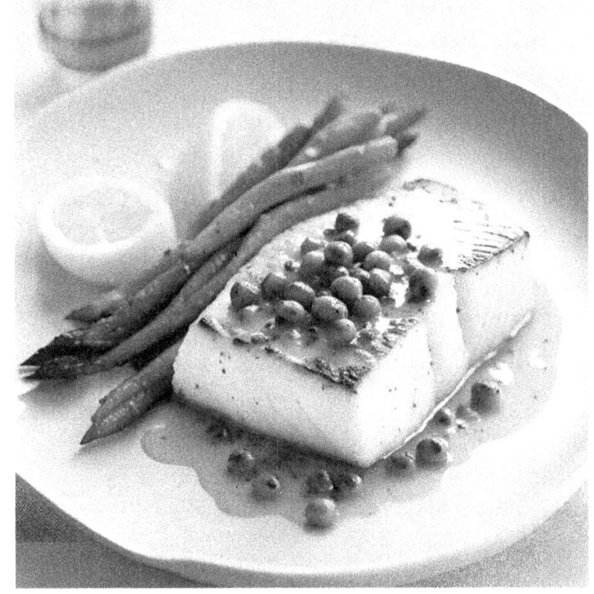

16. Shrimp Scampi with Zucchini Noodles

Ingredients:

- 1 lb large shrimp, peeled and deveined
- 2 tablespoons olive oil
- 4 cloves garlic, minced
- 1/4 teaspoon red pepper flakes (optional)
- 1/4 cup dry white wine
- 2 tablespoons lemon juice
- 1/4 cup unsalted butter
- 4 medium zucchinis, spiralized
- 1/4 cup fresh parsley, chopped
- 1/2 teaspoon sea salt
- 1/4 teaspoon black pepper

Instructions:

1. Heat the olive oil in a large skillet over medium-high heat.
2. Add the shrimp and cook for 2-3 minutes per side, or until pink and opaque. Remove and set aside.
3. In the same skillet, add the garlic and red pepper flakes (if using). Cook for 1 minute until fragrant.
4. Add the white wine and lemon juice, bringing to a simmer.
5. Stir in the butter until melted.
6. Add the zucchini noodles and cook for 2-3 minutes, or until just tender.
7. Return the shrimp to the skillet and toss to combine.
8. Season with sea salt and black pepper.
9. Serve hot, garnished with fresh parsley.

Nutrition Info (per serving):

- Calories: 300
- Carbohydrates: 10g
- Protein: 28g
- Fat: 18g
- Fiber: 3g
- Sugar: 5g

Number of Serves: 4
Cooking Time: 20 minutes

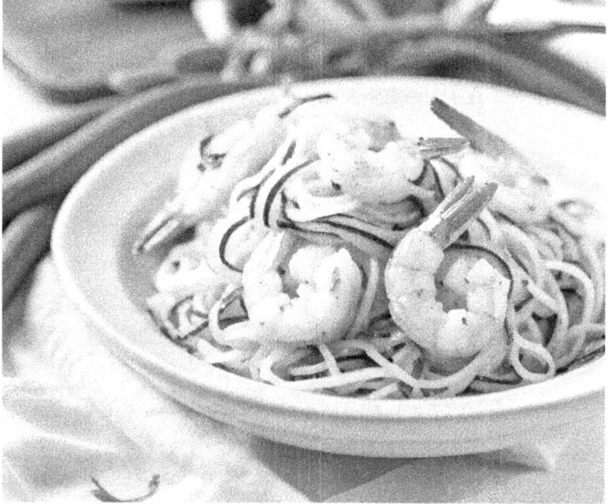

17. Crab Cakes with Lemon Aioli

Ingredients:

- 1 lb lump crab meat
- 1/2 cup whole wheat bread crumbs
- 1/4 cup mayonnaise
- 1 egg, beaten
- 1 tablespoon Dijon mustard
- 1 tablespoon lemon juice
- 1 tablespoon fresh parsley, chopped
- 1/2 teaspoon sea salt
- 1/4 teaspoon black pepper
- 2 tablespoons olive oil (for frying)

For Lemon Aioli:

- 1/2 cup mayonnaise
- 1 tablespoon lemon juice
- 1 teaspoon lemon zest
- 1 clove garlic, minced
- 1/4 teaspoon sea salt

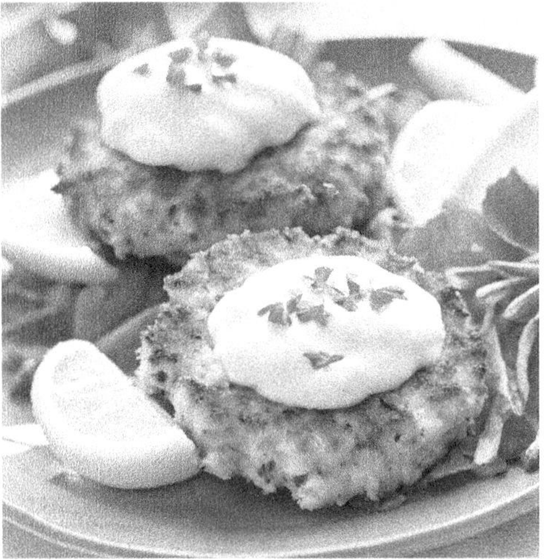

Instructions:

1. In a large bowl, combine the crab meat, bread crumbs, mayonnaise, egg, Dijon mustard, lemon juice, parsley, sea salt, and black pepper. Mix gently until well combined.
2. Form the mixture into 8 patties and refrigerate for 30 minutes to set.
3. Heat olive oil in a large skillet over medium-high heat.
4. Cook the crab cakes for 3-4 minutes per side, or until golden brown and heated through.
5. For the lemon aioli, mix the mayonnaise, lemon juice, lemon zest, garlic, and sea salt in a small bowl.
6. Serve the crab cakes hot with lemon aioli on the side.

Nutrition Info (per serving):

- Calories: 300
- Carbohydrates: 12g
- Protein: 22g
- Fat: 18g
- Fiber: 2g
- Sugar: 1g

Number of Serves: 4

Cooking Time: 40 minutes (including chilling time)

18. Lobster Roll

Ingredients:

- 1 lb cooked lobster meat, chopped
- 1/4 cup mayonnaise
- 1 tablespoon lemon juice
- 1 celery stalk, finely chopped
- 2 tablespoons fresh chives, chopped
- 1/4 teaspoon sea salt
- 1/4 teaspoon black pepper
- 4 whole wheat hot dog buns
- 2 tablespoons butter, melted

Instructions:

1. In a large bowl, combine the lobster meat, mayonnaise, lemon juice, celery, chives, sea salt, and black pepper. Mix until well combined.
2. Brush the hot dog buns with melted butter and toast in a skillet over medium heat until golden brown.
3. Fill each bun with the lobster mixture.
4. Serve immediately.

Nutrition Info (per serving):

- Calories: 350
- Carbohydrates: 30g
- Protein: 22g
- Fat: 18g
- Fiber: 4g
- Sugar: 2g

Number of Serves: 4
Cooking Time: 15 minutes

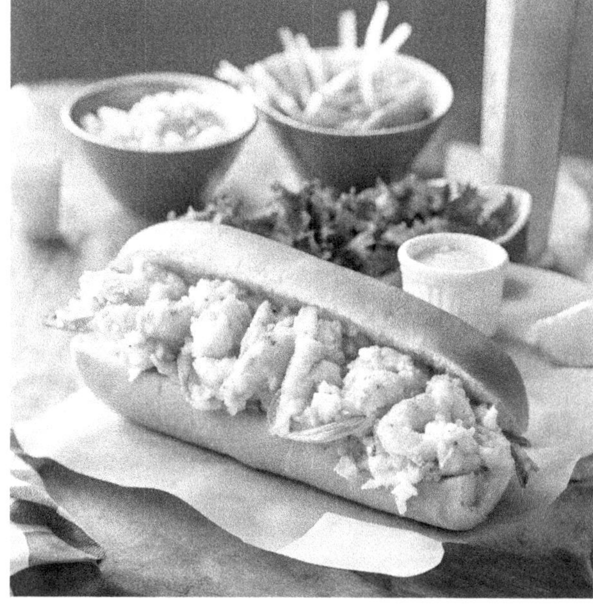

19. Grilled Octopus with Olives and Oregano

Ingredients:

- 2 lbs octopus, cleaned
- 4 tablespoons olive oil, divided
- 1 lemon, juiced
- 2 cloves garlic, minced
- 1/4 cup Kalamata olives, pitted and sliced
- 1 tablespoon fresh oregano, chopped
- 1/2 teaspoon sea salt
- 1/4 teaspoon black pepper

Instructions:

1. Bring a large pot of water to a boil and cook the octopus for 45-60 minutes, or until tender. Remove and let cool.
2. Preheat the grill to medium-high heat.
3. Cut the octopus into serving-sized pieces and toss with 2 tablespoons of olive oil, lemon juice, garlic, sea salt, and black pepper.
4. Grill the octopus for 4-5 minutes per side, until slightly charred.
5. In a small bowl, mix the remaining olive oil, olives, and oregano.
6. Serve the grilled octopus topped with the olive and oregano mixture.

Nutrition Info (per serving):

- Calories: 300
- Carbohydrates: 6g
- Protein: 28g
- Fat: 18g
- Fiber: 2g
- Sugar: 0g

Number of Serves: 4
Cooking Time: 1 hour 15 minutes

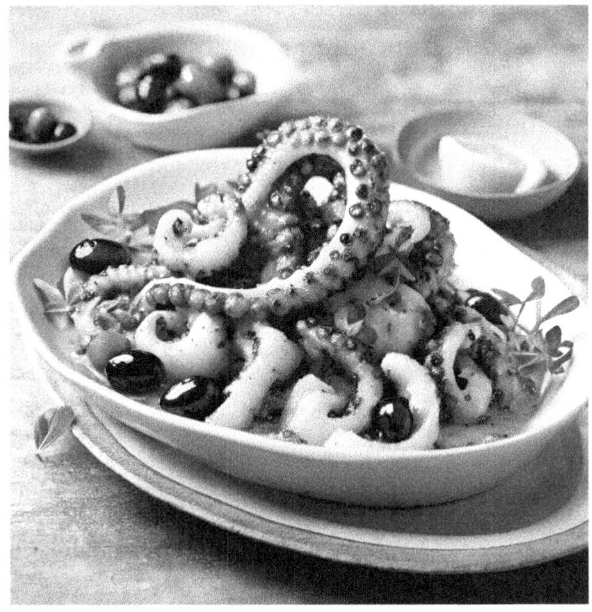

20. Seafood Paella

Ingredients:

- 1/2 lb shrimp, peeled and deveined
- 1/2 lb mussels, cleaned
- 1/2 lb squid, sliced into rings
- 2 tablespoons olive oil
- 1 large onion, diced
- 3 cloves garlic, minced
- 1 red bell pepper, diced
- 1 cup short-grain rice
- 1/2 teaspoon saffron threads, soaked in 2 tablespoons warm water
- 4 cups fish stock (low sodium)
- 1 cup diced tomatoes
- 1 teaspoon smoked paprika
- 1/2 teaspoon sea salt
- 1/4 teaspoon black pepper
- 1/4 cup fresh parsley, chopped
- 1 lemon, cut into wedges

Instructions:

1. Heat the olive oil in a large, deep skillet or paella pan over medium heat.
2. Add the onion, garlic, and red bell pepper, sautéing for 5-7 minutes until softened.
3. Stir in the rice and cook for 1-2 minutes, until lightly toasted.
4. Add the saffron water, fish stock, diced tomatoes, smoked paprika, sea salt, and black pepper. Bring to a simmer.
5. Arrange the shrimp, mussels, and squid over the rice. Cover and cook for 15-20 minutes, or until the rice is tender and the seafood is cooked through.
6. Remove from heat and let rest for 5 minutes.
7. Garnish with fresh parsley and lemon wedges before serving.

Nutrition Info (per serving):

- Calories: 400
- Carbohydrates: 40g
- Protein: 28g
- Fat: 12g
- Fiber: 4g
- Sugar: 6g

Number of Serves: 4

Cooking Time: 35 minutes

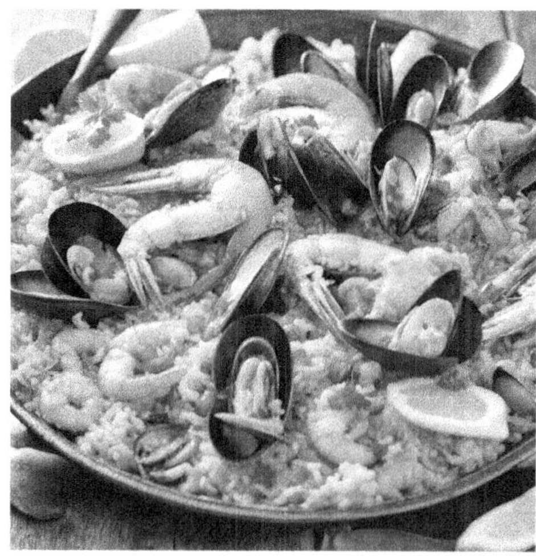

21. Oysters Rockefeller

Ingredients:

- 12 fresh oysters, shucked
- 2 tablespoons olive oil
- 1/2 cup finely chopped spinach
- 1/4 cup finely chopped parsley
- 2 cloves garlic, minced
- 1/4 cup grated Parmesan cheese
- 2 tablespoons bread crumbs (whole wheat)
- 2 tablespoons lemon juice
- 1/4 teaspoon sea salt
- 1/4 teaspoon black pepper

Instructions:

1. Preheat the oven to 450°F (230°C).
2. In a skillet, heat the olive oil over medium heat.
3. Add the spinach, parsley, and garlic. Cook for 3-4 minutes until the spinach is wilted.
4. Remove from heat and stir in the Parmesan cheese, bread crumbs, lemon juice, sea salt, and black pepper.
5. **Spoon the spinach mixture over each oyster.**
6. Place the oysters on a baking sheet and bake for 10-12 minutes, or until the topping is golden and the oysters are cooked through.
7. Serve immediately.

Nutrition Info (per serving):

- Calories: 150
- Carbohydrates: 5g
- Protein: 12g
- Fat: 8g
- Fiber: 1g
- Sugar: 1g

Number of Serves: 4

Cooking Time: 20 minutes

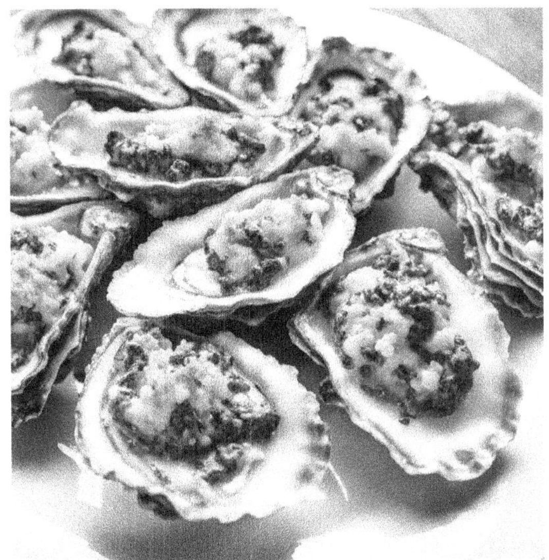

22. Prawn Risotto

Ingredients:

- 1 lb large prawns, peeled and deveined
- 2 tablespoons olive oil
- 1 large onion, diced
- 2 cloves garlic, minced
- 1 cup Arborio rice
- 1/2 cup dry white wine
- 4 cups low sodium chicken broth, warmed
- 1/4 cup grated Parmesan cheese
- 2 tablespoons fresh parsley, chopped
- 1 tablespoon lemon juice
- 1/2 teaspoon sea salt
- 1/4 teaspoon black pepper

Instructions:

1. Heat the olive oil in a large skillet over medium heat.
2. Add the onion and garlic, sautéing for 3-4 minutes until softened.
3. Stir in the Arborio rice and cook for 2-3 minutes, until lightly toasted.
4. Add the white wine and cook until mostly absorbed.
5. Gradually add the warm chicken broth, one ladle at a time, stirring constantly and allowing the liquid to be absorbed before adding more. This process should take about 20 minutes.
6. When the rice is almost cooked, stir in the prawns and cook for 3-4 minutes, or until the prawns are pink and opaque.
7. Stir in the Parmesan cheese, parsley, lemon juice, sea salt, and black pepper.
8. Serve hot.

Nutrition Info (per serving):

- Calories: 350
- Carbohydrates: 40g
- Protein: 25g
- Fat: 10g
- Fiber: 2g
- Sugar: 3g

Number of Serves: 4

Cooking Time: 30 minutes

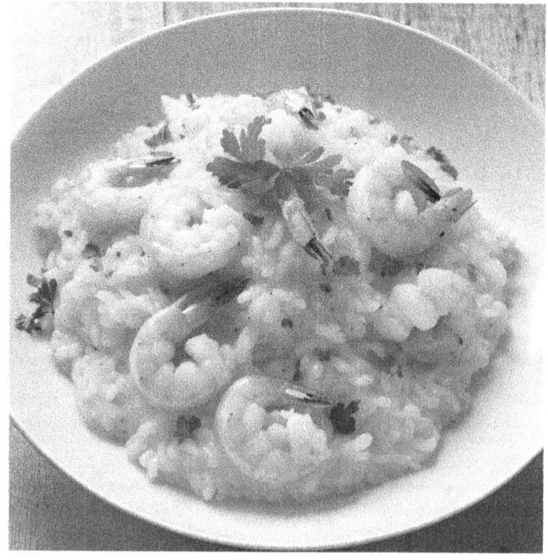

23. Spicy Calamari Stir Fry

Ingredients:

- 1 lb calamari, cleaned and cut into rings
- 2 tablespoons olive oil
- 1 red bell pepper, sliced
- 1 yellow bell pepper, sliced
- 1 small onion, sliced
- 3 cloves garlic, minced
- 1 tablespoon ginger, minced
- 1 red chili, sliced
- 2 tablespoons soy sauce (low sodium)
- 1 tablespoon rice vinegar
- 1 tablespoon honey or maple syrup
- 1/4 teaspoon sea salt
- 1/4 teaspoon black pepper
- 2 green onions, chopped (for garnish)

Instructions:

1. Heat the olive oil in a large skillet or wok over medium-high heat.
2. Add the onion, garlic, ginger, and chili. Stir-fry for 2-3 minutes until fragrant.
3. Add the red and yellow bell peppers and stir-fry for another 3-4 minutes until tender.
4. Add the calamari rings and stir-fry for 2-3 minutes until just cooked through.
5. Stir in the soy sauce, rice vinegar, honey or maple syrup, sea salt, and black pepper. Cook for another minute.
6. Garnish with chopped green onions and serve immediately.

Nutrition Info (per serving):

- Calories: 220
- Carbohydrates: 15g
- Protein: 25g
- Fat: 8g
- Fiber: 3g
- Sugar: 6g

Number of Serves: 4
Cooking Time: 15 minutes

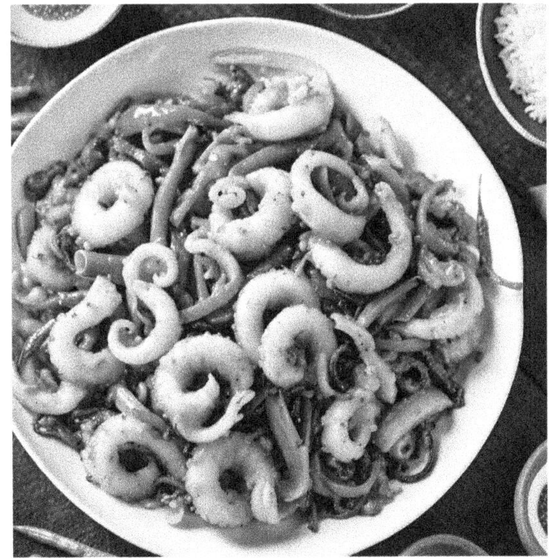

24. Steamed Clams with Garlic Butter

Ingredients:

- 2 lbs fresh clams, cleaned
- 2 tablespoons olive oil
- 4 cloves garlic, minced
- 1/2 cup dry white wine
- 1/4 cup unsalted butter
- 1/4 cup fresh parsley, chopped
- 1 lemon, juiced
- 1/2 teaspoon sea salt
- 1/4 teaspoon black pepper

Instructions:

1. Heat the olive oil in a large pot over medium heat.
2. Add the garlic and cook for 1-2 minutes until fragrant.
3. Add the white wine and bring to a simmer.
4. Add the clams, cover the pot, and steam for 5-7 minutes, or until the clams open. Discard any that do not open.
5. Remove the clams with a slotted spoon and set aside.
6. Stir in the butter, parsley, lemon juice, sea salt, and black pepper into the pot. Cook until the butter is melted and the sauce is well combined.
7. Pour the garlic butter sauce over the clams and serve hot.

Nutrition Info (per serving):

- Calories: 250
- Carbohydrates: 10g
- Protein: 20g
- Fat: 12g
- Fiber: 1g
- Sugar: 1g

Number of Serves: 4

Cooking Time: 15 minutes

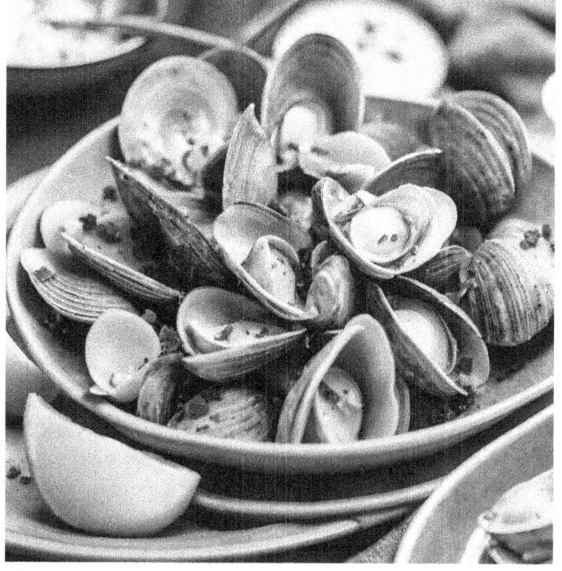

25. Seafood Gumbo

Ingredients:

- 1/2 lb shrimp, peeled and deveined
- 1/2 lb crab meat
- 1/2 lb scallops
- 2 tablespoons olive oil
- 1 large onion, diced
- 1 green bell pepper, diced
- 2 celery stalks, diced
- 3 cloves garlic, minced
- 1 (14 oz) can diced tomatoes
- 4 cups low sodium chicken broth
- 1/4 cup whole wheat flour
- 1 tablespoon Cajun seasoning
- 1/2 teaspoon sea salt
- 1/4 teaspoon black pepper
- 2 bay leaves
- 1/2 teaspoon dried thyme
- 1/4 cup fresh parsley, chopped
- Cooked brown rice, for serving

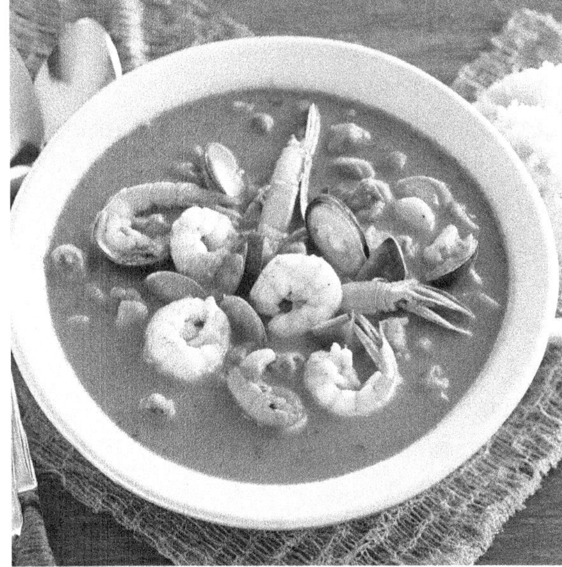

Instructions:

1. In a large pot, heat the olive oil over medium heat.
2. Add the flour and cook, stirring constantly, for 5-7 minutes until it turns a deep brown color to make a roux.
3. Add the onion, bell pepper, celery, and garlic. Cook for 5-7 minutes until softened.
4. Stir in the diced tomatoes, chicken broth, Cajun seasoning, sea salt, black pepper, bay leaves, and thyme. Bring to a simmer.
5. Add the shrimp, crab meat, and scallops. Cook for 10-15 minutes, or until the seafood is cooked through.
6. Remove the bay leaves before serving.
7. Serve the gumbo hot over cooked brown rice, garnished with fresh parsley.

Nutrition Info (per serving):

- Calories: 350
- Carbohydrates: 30g
- Protein: 28g
- Fat: 12g
- Fiber: 4g
- Sugar: 6g

Number of Serves: 4

Cooking Time: 40 minutes

26. Fried Squid Rings with Aioli

Ingredients:

- 1 lb squid, cleaned and cut into rings
- 1 cup whole wheat flour
- 1/2 teaspoon sea salt
- 1/4 teaspoon black pepper
- 1/4 teaspoon paprika
- 2 eggs, beaten
- 1/2 cup whole wheat bread crumbs
- 2 cups olive oil (for frying)

For Aioli:

- 1/2 cup mayonnaise
- 1 tablespoon lemon juice
- 1 clove garlic, minced
- 1/4 teaspoon sea salt

Instructions:

1. In a shallow bowl, mix the flour, sea salt, black pepper, and paprika.
2. In another shallow bowl, place the beaten eggs.
3. In a third shallow bowl, place the bread crumbs.
4. Dredge the squid rings in the flour mixture, dip in the beaten eggs, and then coat with bread crumbs.
5. Heat the olive oil in a large skillet over medium-high heat.
6. Fry the squid rings in batches for 2-3 minutes per side, or until golden brown and crispy. Drain on paper towels.
7. For the aioli, mix the mayonnaise, lemon juice, garlic, and sea salt in a small bowl.
8. Serve the fried squid rings hot with aioli on the side.

Nutrition Info (per serving):

- Calories: 350
- Carbohydrates: 20g
- Protein: 22g
- Fat: 20g
- Fiber: 3g
- Sugar: 1g

Number of Serves: 4
Cooking Time: 20 minutes

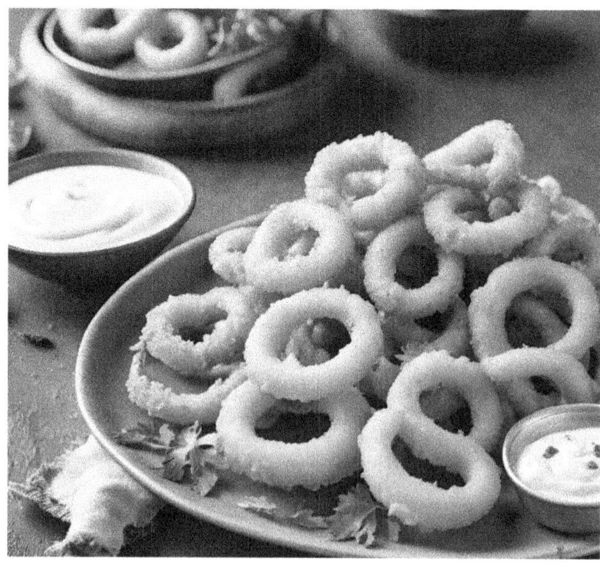

27. Crayfish Boil

Ingredients:

- 2 lbs crayfish, cleaned
- 4 ears corn, cut into thirds
- 4 red potatoes, halved
- 1 large onion, quartered
- 3 cloves garlic, smashed
- 2 lemons, halved
- 1/4 cup Old Bay seasoning
- 1 tablespoon sea salt
- 2 tablespoons olive oil

Instructions:

1. Fill a large pot with water and add the Old Bay seasoning, sea salt, garlic, and lemons. Bring to a boil.
2. Add the potatoes and cook for 10 minutes.
3. Add the corn and onion, cooking for another 5 minutes.
4. Add the crayfish and cook for an additional 5-7 minutes, or until the crayfish are bright red and cooked through.
5. Drain the crayfish and vegetables, then toss with olive oil.
6. Serve hot with lemon wedges.

Nutrition Info (per serving):

- Calories: 350
- Carbohydrates: 40g
- Protein: 25g
- Fat: 8g
- Fiber: 6g
- Sugar: 4g

Number of Serves: 4
Cooking Time: 30 minutes

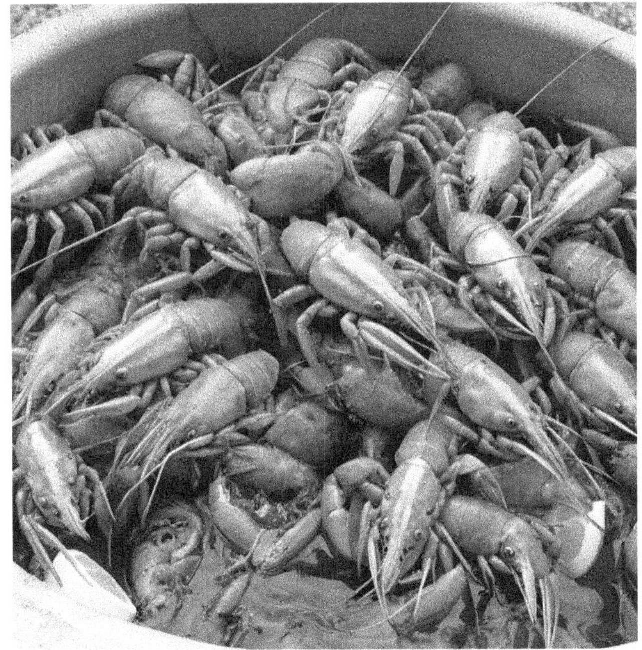

28. Seafood Chowder

Ingredients:

- 1/2 lb shrimp, peeled and deveined
- 1/2 lb cod, cut into chunks
- 1/2 lb clams, cleaned
- 2 tablespoons olive oil
- 1 large onion, diced
- 2 celery stalks, diced
- 3 cloves garlic, minced
- 2 large potatoes, peeled and diced
- 4 cups low sodium chicken broth
- 1 cup almond milk (unsweetened)
- 1/4 cup whole wheat flour
- 1 teaspoon dried thyme
- 1/2 teaspoon sea salt
- 1/4 teaspoon black pepper
- 1/4 cup fresh parsley, chopped

Instructions:

1. Heat the olive oil in a large pot over medium heat.
2. Add the onion, celery, and garlic. Sauté for 5-7 minutes until softened.
3. Stir in the flour and cook for another 1-2 minutes.
4. Add the chicken broth, almond milk, potatoes, thyme, sea salt, and black pepper. Bring to a simmer and cook for 15 minutes, or until the potatoes are tender.
5. Add the shrimp, cod, and clams. Cook for 5-7 minutes, or until the seafood is cooked through and the clams have opened.
6. Remove any clams that did not open.
7. Serve hot, garnished with fresh parsley.

Nutrition Info (per serving):

- Calories: 300
- Carbohydrates: 30g
- Protein: 25g
- Fat: 10g
- Fiber: 4g
- Sugar: 3g

Number of Serves: 4

Cooking Time: 30 minutes

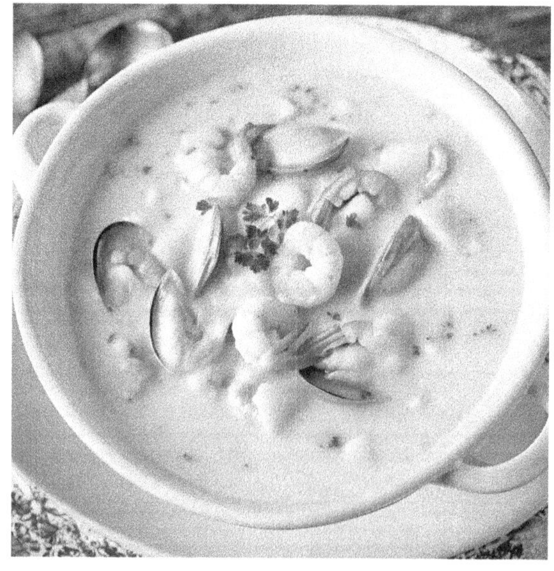

Poultry Recipes

1. Grilled Chicken Breast with Herbed Quinoa
Ingredients:
- 4 boneless, skinless chicken breasts
- 2 tablespoons olive oil
- 2 cloves garlic, minced
- 1 teaspoon dried thyme
- 1 teaspoon dried rosemary
- 1 teaspoon sea salt
- 1/2 teaspoon black pepper
- 1 cup quinoa
- 2 cups low sodium chicken broth
- 1/4 cup fresh parsley, chopped
- 1/4 cup fresh mint, chopped
- 1 lemon, juiced and zested

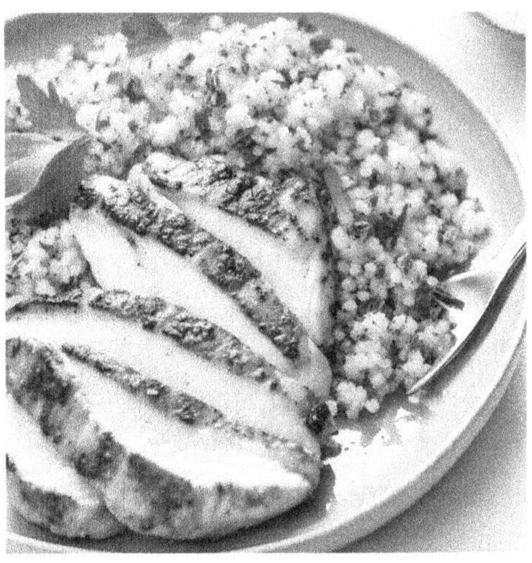

Instructions:
1. Preheat the grill to medium-high heat.
2. In a small bowl, mix the olive oil, garlic, thyme, rosemary, sea salt, and black pepper. Rub the mixture evenly over the chicken breasts.
3. Grill the chicken for 6-8 minutes per side, or until the internal temperature reaches 165°F (74°C).
4. While the chicken is grilling, rinse the quinoa under cold water.
5. In a medium saucepan, bring the chicken broth to a boil. Add the quinoa, reduce heat to low, cover, and simmer for 15 minutes, or until the quinoa is tender and the liquid is absorbed.
6. Remove the quinoa from heat and stir in the fresh parsley, mint, lemon juice, and lemon zest.
7. Serve the grilled chicken breast on a bed of herbed quinoa.

Nutrition Info (per serving):
- Calories: 350
- Carbohydrates: 25g
- Protein: 35g
- Fat: 12g
- Fiber: 3g
- Sugar: 1g

Number of Serves: 4
Cooking Time: 30 minutes

2. Chicken and Vegetable Stir-Fry

Ingredients:

- 1 lb boneless, skinless chicken breasts, thinly sliced
- 2 tablespoons olive oil
- 2 cloves garlic, minced
- 1 tablespoon ginger, minced
- 1 red bell pepper, sliced
- 1 yellow bell pepper, sliced
- 1 small broccoli head, cut into florets
- 1 carrot, julienned
- 1/4 cup low sodium soy sauce
- 1 tablespoon rice vinegar
- 1 tablespoon honey or maple syrup
- 1/4 teaspoon sea salt
- 1/4 teaspoon black pepper
- 2 green onions, chopped (for garnish)

Instructions:

1. Heat 1 tablespoon of olive oil in a large skillet or wok over medium-high heat.
2. Add the sliced chicken and cook for 5-7 minutes until browned and cooked through. Remove from the skillet and set aside.
3. In the same skillet, add the remaining olive oil, garlic, and ginger. Sauté for 1-2 minutes until fragrant.
4. Add the bell peppers, broccoli, and carrot. Stir-fry for 5-7 minutes until the vegetables are tender-crisp.
5. Return the chicken to the skillet.
6. In a small bowl, mix the soy sauce, rice vinegar, honey or maple syrup, sea salt, and black pepper.
7. Pour the sauce over the chicken and vegetables, stirring to coat evenly. Cook for an additional 2-3 minutes until heated through.
8. Serve hot, garnished with chopped green onions.

Nutrition Info (per serving):

- Calories: 300
- Carbohydrates: 20g
- Protein: 30g
- Fat: 12g
- Fiber: 4g
- Sugar: 8g

Number of Serves: 4

Cooking Time: 20 minutes

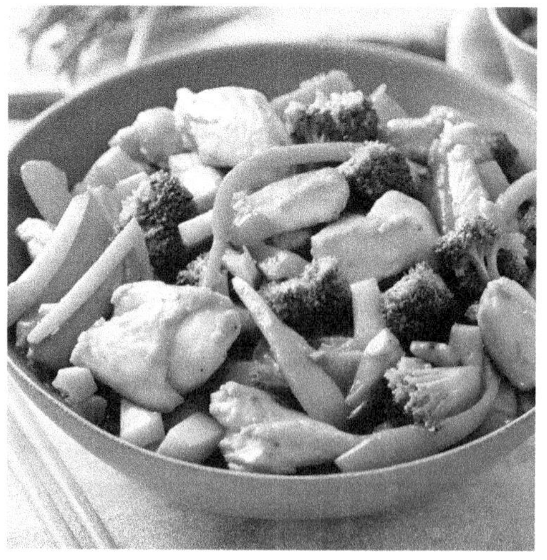

3. Baked Lemon Pepper Chicken

Ingredients:

- 4 boneless, skinless chicken breasts
- 2 tablespoons olive oil
- 1 lemon, sliced
- 1 teaspoon lemon zest
- 2 tablespoons lemon juice
- 1 teaspoon freshly ground black pepper
- 1 teaspoon sea salt
- 2 cloves garlic, minced
- 1 teaspoon dried thyme

Instructions:

1. Preheat the oven to 375°F (190°C).
2. In a small bowl, mix the olive oil, lemon zest, lemon juice, black pepper, sea salt, garlic, and thyme.
3. Rub the mixture evenly over the chicken breasts.
4. Place the chicken breasts in a baking dish and top with lemon slices.
5. Bake for 25-30 minutes, or until the internal temperature reaches 165°F (74°C) and the chicken is cooked through.
6. Serve hot, garnished with additional lemon slices if desired.

Nutrition Info (per serving):

- Calories: 250
- Carbohydrates: 2g
- Protein: 30g
- Fat: 14g
- Fiber: 1g
- Sugar: 1g

Number of Serves: 4
Cooking Time: 30 minutes

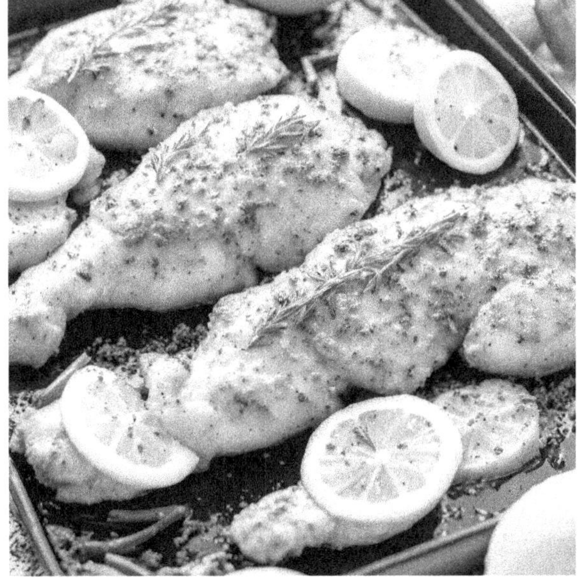

4. Moroccan Chicken Tagine

Ingredients:

- 1 1/2 lbs boneless, skinless chicken thighs, cut into chunks
- 2 tablespoons olive oil
- 1 large onion, diced
- 3 cloves garlic, minced
- 1 tablespoon ginger, minced
- 1 teaspoon ground cumin
- 1 teaspoon ground coriander
- 1 teaspoon ground cinnamon
- 1/2 teaspoon ground turmeric
- 1/2 teaspoon sea salt
- 1/4 teaspoon black pepper
- 1/4 teaspoon cayenne pepper (optional)
- 1 (14 oz) can diced tomatoes
- 1 cup low sodium chicken broth
- 1/2 cup dried apricots, chopped
- 1/4 cup green olives, pitted and sliced
- 1/4 cup fresh cilantro, chopped
- 1/4 cup fresh parsley, chopped
- Cooked couscous, for serving

Instructions:

1. Heat the olive oil in a large pot or tagine over medium heat.
2. Add the onion, garlic, and ginger. Sauté for 5-7 minutes until softened.
3. Stir in the cumin, coriander, cinnamon, turmeric, sea salt, black pepper, and cayenne pepper (if using). Cook for 1-2 minutes until fragrant.
4. Add the chicken chunks and cook for 5-7 minutes until browned on all sides.
5. Stir in the diced tomatoes, chicken broth, dried apricots, and green olives.
6. Bring to a simmer, then reduce heat to low and cover. Cook for 30-35 minutes, or until the chicken is cooked through and tender.
7. Stir in the fresh cilantro and parsley.
8. Serve the Moroccan chicken tagine hot over cooked couscous.

Nutrition Info (per serving):

- Calories: 400
- Carbohydrates: 25g
- Protein: 30g
- Fat: 18g
- Fiber: 4g
- Sugar: 10g

Number of Serves: 4

Cooking Time: 45 minutes

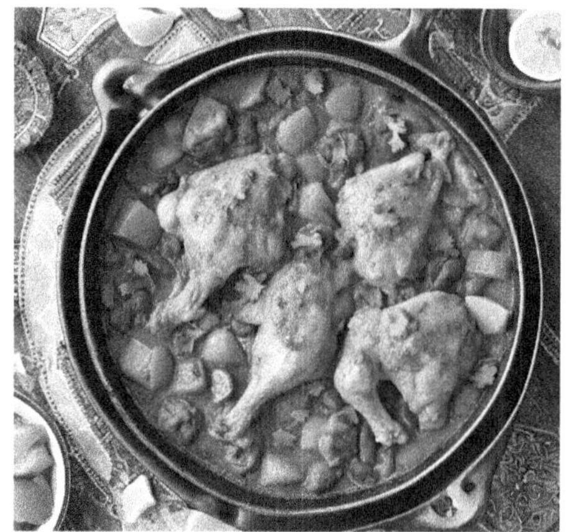

5. Spinach and Feta Stuffed Chicken

Ingredients:

- 4 boneless, skinless chicken breasts
- 2 tablespoons olive oil
- 2 cups fresh spinach, chopped
- 1/2 cup feta cheese, crumbled
- 2 cloves garlic, minced
- 1 teaspoon dried oregano
- 1/2 teaspoon sea salt
- 1/4 teaspoon black pepper
- 1 lemon, sliced (for garnish)

Instructions:

1. Preheat the oven to 375°F (190°C).
2. In a skillet, heat 1 tablespoon of olive oil over medium heat. Add the garlic and sauté for 1 minute until fragrant.
3. Add the chopped spinach and cook for 2-3 minutes until wilted. Remove from heat and let cool slightly.
4. Stir in the feta cheese, oregano, sea salt, and black pepper.
5. Cut a pocket into each chicken breast and stuff with the spinach and feta mixture.
6. Secure the openings with toothpicks.
7. In an oven-safe skillet, heat the remaining olive oil over medium-high heat. Sear the stuffed chicken breasts for 2-3 minutes per side until golden brown.
8. Transfer the skillet to the oven and bake for 20-25 minutes, or until the chicken is cooked through and the internal temperature reaches 165°F (74°C).
9. Serve hot, garnished with lemon slices.

Nutrition Info (per serving):

- Calories: 350
- Carbohydrates: 3g
- Protein: 35g
- Fat: 20g
- Fiber: 1g
- Sugar: 1g

Number of Serves: 4
Cooking Time: 35 minutes

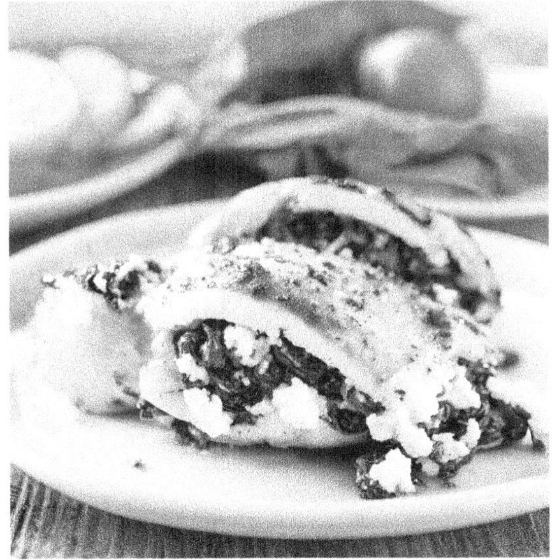

6. BBQ Chicken Pizza

Ingredients:
- 1 whole wheat pizza crust
- 1/2 cup BBQ sauce (low sugar)
- 1 cup cooked chicken breast, shredded
- 1/2 red onion, thinly sliced
- 1 cup mozzarella cheese, shredded
- 1/4 cup fresh cilantro, chopped

Instructions:
1. Preheat the oven to 425°F (220°C).
2. Spread the BBQ sauce evenly over the pizza crust.
3. Top with shredded chicken, red onion slices, and mozzarella cheese.
4. Bake for 12-15 minutes, or until the cheese is melted and bubbly.
5. Remove from the oven and sprinkle with fresh cilantro.
6. Slice and serve hot.

Nutrition Info (per serving):
- Calories: 350
- Carbohydrates: 40g
- Protein: 25g
- Fat: 12g
- Fiber: 4g
- Sugar: 8g

Number of Serves: 4
Cooking Time: 20 minutes

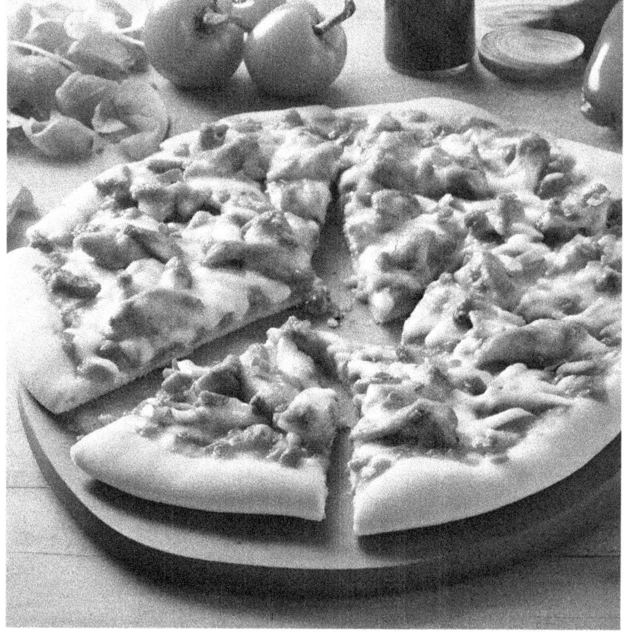

7. Thai Chicken Coconut Curry

Ingredients:

- 1 lb boneless, skinless chicken thighs, cut into chunks
- 2 tablespoons olive oil
- 1 large onion, diced
- 3 cloves garlic, minced
- 1 tablespoon ginger, minced
- 1 red bell pepper, sliced
- 1 yellow bell pepper, sliced
- 2 tablespoons red curry paste
- 1 (14 oz) can coconut milk
- 1 cup low sodium chicken broth
- 1 tablespoon fish sauce
- 1 tablespoon lime juice
- 1 teaspoon sea salt
- 1/4 teaspoon black pepper
- 1/4 cup fresh cilantro, chopped
- Cooked brown rice, for serving

Instructions:

1. Heat the olive oil in a large pot over medium heat.
2. Add the onion, garlic, and ginger. Sauté for 3-4 minutes until softened.
3. Stir in the red curry paste and cook for another minute until fragrant.
4. Add the chicken chunks and cook for 5-7 minutes until browned on all sides.
5. Stir in the bell peppers, coconut milk, chicken broth, fish sauce, lime juice, sea salt, and black pepper. Bring to a simmer.
6. Cook for 15-20 minutes, or until the chicken is cooked through and the sauce has thickened.
7. Serve the Thai chicken coconut curry hot over cooked brown rice, garnished with fresh cilantro.

Nutrition Info (per serving):

- Calories: 400
- Carbohydrates: 30g
- Protein: 28g
- Fat: 20g
- Fiber: 4g
- Sugar: 6g

Number of Serves: 4

Cooking Time: 30 minutes

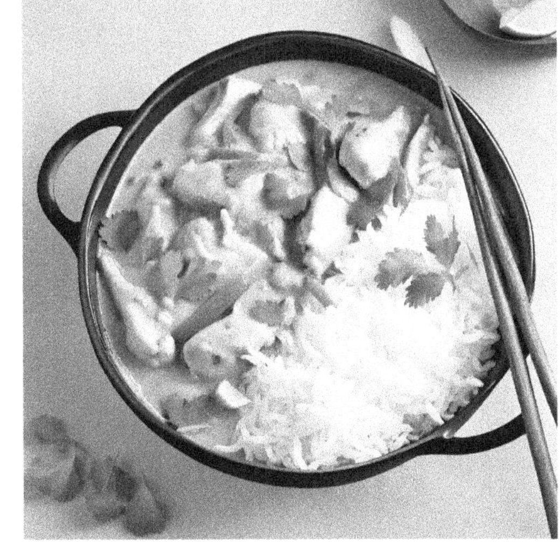

8. Chicken Piccata with Capers

Ingredients:

- 4 boneless, skinless chicken breasts
- 1/2 cup whole wheat flour
- 1/2 teaspoon sea salt
- 1/4 teaspoon black pepper
- 2 tablespoons olive oil
- 1/4 cup lemon juice
- 1/2 cup low sodium chicken broth
- 1/4 cup capers, rinsed
- 1/4 cup fresh parsley, chopped

Instructions:

1. Season the chicken breasts with sea salt and black pepper.
2. Dredge the chicken breasts in whole wheat flour, shaking off any excess.
3. Heat the olive oil in a large skillet over medium-high heat.
4. Cook the chicken breasts for 3-4 minutes per side, or until golden brown and cooked through. Remove from the skillet and set aside.
5. In the same skillet, add the lemon juice, chicken broth, and capers. Bring to a simmer, scraping up any browned bits from the bottom of the skillet.
6. Return the chicken to the skillet and simmer for 5 minutes, or until heated through.
7. Serve hot, garnished with fresh parsley.

Nutrition Info (per serving):

- Calories: 300
- Carbohydrates: 12g
- Protein: 30g
- Fat: 14g
- Fiber: 2g
- Sugar: 1g

Number of Serves: 4

Cooking Time: 20 minutes

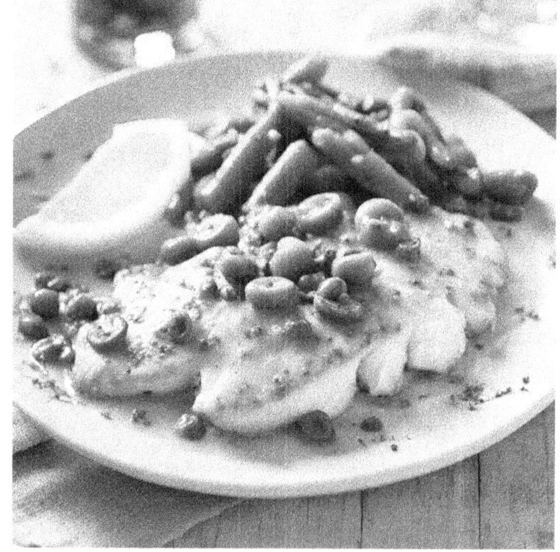

9. Chicken Fajitas

Ingredients:

- 1 lb boneless, skinless chicken breasts, thinly sliced
- 2 tablespoons olive oil
- 1 red bell pepper, sliced
- 1 green bell pepper, sliced
- 1 yellow bell pepper, sliced
- 1 large onion, sliced
- 2 cloves garlic, minced
- 1 teaspoon ground cumin
- 1 teaspoon chili powder
- 1/2 teaspoon sea salt
- 1/4 teaspoon black pepper
- 8 whole wheat tortillas
- Fresh cilantro, chopped (for garnish)
- Lime wedges (for serving)

Instructions:

1. Heat 1 tablespoon of olive oil in a large skillet over medium-high heat.
2. Add the chicken slices and cook for 5-7 minutes until browned and cooked through. Remove from the skillet and set aside.
3. In the same skillet, add the remaining olive oil, bell peppers, onion, and garlic. Sauté for 5-7 minutes until tender.
4. Return the chicken to the skillet and stir in the cumin, chili powder, sea salt, and black pepper. Cook for another 2-3 minutes until heated through.
5. Warm the tortillas in a dry skillet or in the oven.
6. Serve the chicken and vegetable mixture in the tortillas, garnished with fresh cilantro and lime wedges.

Nutrition Info (per serving):

- Calories: 300
- Carbohydrates: 35g
- Protein: 25g
- Fat: 10g
- Fiber: 6g
- Sugar: 3g

Number of Serves: 4

Cooking Time: 20 minutes

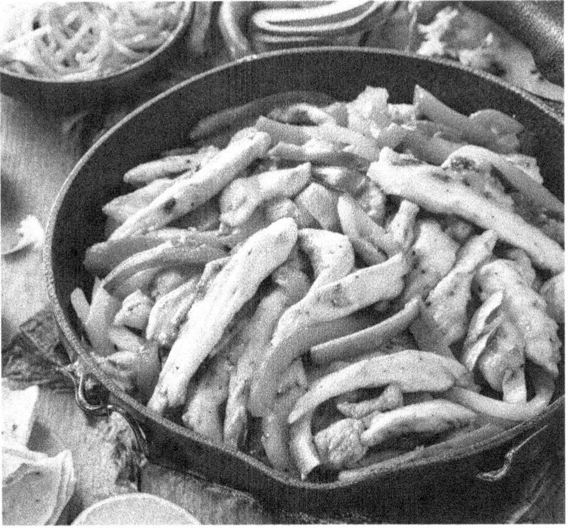

10. Roast Chicken with Root Vegetables

Ingredients:

- 1 whole chicken (about 4 lbs)
- 2 tablespoons olive oil
- 2 cloves garlic, minced
- 1 tablespoon fresh rosemary, chopped
- 1 tablespoon fresh thyme, chopped
- 1 teaspoon sea salt
- 1/2 teaspoon black pepper
- 4 large carrots, peeled and cut into chunks
- 4 parsnips, peeled and cut into chunks
- 2 large potatoes, cut into chunks
- 1 large onion, cut into wedges
- 1 lemon, halved

Instructions:

1. Preheat the oven to 375°F (190°C).
2. In a small bowl, mix the olive oil, garlic, rosemary, thyme, sea salt, and black pepper.
3. Rub the mixture all over the chicken, including under the skin.
4. Place the chicken in a roasting pan and surround it with the carrots, parsnips, potatoes, and onion.
5. Squeeze the lemon halves over the chicken and vegetables, then place the lemon halves in the roasting pan.
6. Roast for 1 1/2 to 2 hours, or until the internal temperature of the chicken reaches 165°F (74°C) and the vegetables are tender.
7. Let the chicken rest for 10 minutes before carving.
8. Serve the roast chicken with the roasted root vegetables.

Nutrition Info (per serving):

- Calories: 500
- Carbohydrates: 40g
- Protein: 40g
- Fat: 20g
- Fiber: 8g
- Sugar: 8g

Number of Serves: 6

Cooking Time: 2 hours

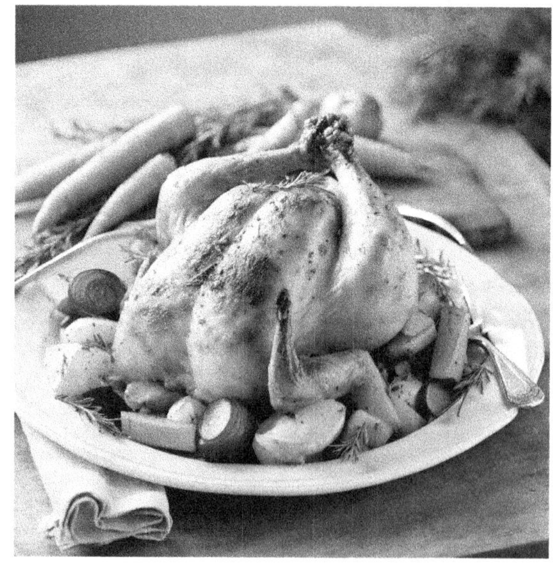

11. Chicken Paella

Ingredients:

- 1 lb boneless, skinless chicken thighs, cut into chunks
- 2 tablespoons olive oil
- 1 large onion, diced
- 3 cloves garlic, minced
- 1 red bell pepper, diced
- 1 yellow bell pepper, diced
- 1 cup short-grain rice
- 1/2 teaspoon saffron threads, soaked in 2 tablespoons warm water
- 4 cups low sodium chicken broth
- 1 (14 oz) can diced tomatoes
- 1 teaspoon smoked paprika
- 1/2 teaspoon sea salt
- 1/4 teaspoon black pepper
- 1/2 cup frozen peas
- 1/4 cup fresh parsley, chopped
- Lemon wedges, for serving

Instructions:

1. Heat the olive oil in a large, deep skillet or paella pan over medium heat.
2. Add the chicken and cook for 5-7 minutes until browned on all sides. Remove and set aside.
3. In the same pan, add the onion, garlic, and bell peppers. Sauté for 5-7 minutes until softened.
4. Stir in the rice and cook for 1-2 minutes until lightly toasted.
5. Add the saffron water, chicken broth, diced tomatoes, smoked paprika, sea salt, and black pepper. Bring to a simmer.
6. Return the chicken to the pan and arrange it evenly over the rice. Cover and cook for 20 minutes.
7. Stir in the frozen peas and cook for an additional 5 minutes, or until the rice is tender and the liquid is absorbed.
8. Serve hot, garnished with fresh parsley and lemon wedges.

Nutrition Info (per serving):

- Calories: 400
- Carbohydrates: 40g
- Protein: 28g
- Fat: 15g
- Fiber: 5g
- Sugar: 6g

Number of Serves: 4
Cooking Time: 35 minutes

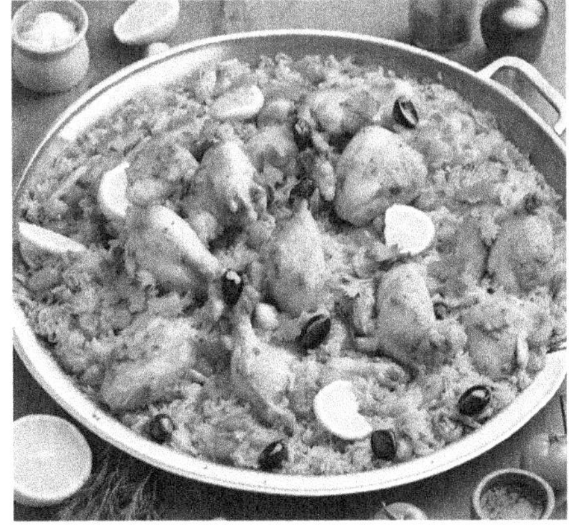

12. Buffalo Chicken Wrap

Ingredients:

- 1 lb boneless, skinless chicken breasts, cut into strips
- 2 tablespoons olive oil
- 1/4 cup hot sauce (POTS-friendly)
- 1/4 cup Greek yogurt (unsweetened)
- 1 teaspoon garlic powder
- 1/2 teaspoon sea salt
- 1/4 teaspoon black pepper
- 4 whole wheat tortillas
- 1 cup shredded lettuce
- 1 cup shredded carrots
- 1/2 cup diced celery
- 1/2 cup crumbled blue cheese (optional)

Instructions:

1. Heat the olive oil in a large skillet over medium-high heat.
2. Add the chicken strips and cook for 5-7 minutes, or until cooked through and lightly browned.
3. In a small bowl, mix the hot sauce, Greek yogurt, garlic powder, sea salt, and black pepper.
4. Toss the cooked chicken in the hot sauce mixture until well coated.
5. Warm the tortillas in a dry skillet or microwave.
6. Divide the chicken among the tortillas and top with shredded lettuce, carrots, celery, and crumbled blue cheese (if using).
7. Wrap the tortillas tightly and serve immediately.

Nutrition Info (per serving):

- Calories: 350
- Carbohydrates: 30g
- Protein: 28g
- Fat: 14g
- Fiber: 6g
- Sugar: 2g

Number of Serves: 4

Cooking Time: 20 minutes

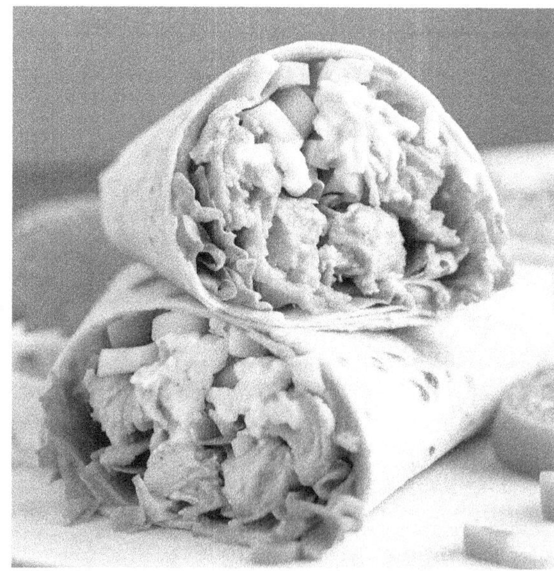

13. Chicken and Broccoli Alfredo

Ingredients:

- 1 lb boneless, skinless chicken breasts, cut into strips
- 2 tablespoons olive oil
- 2 cups broccoli florets
- 3 cloves garlic, minced
- 1 cup unsweetened almond milk
- 1 cup low sodium chicken broth
- 1/2 cup grated Parmesan cheese
- 1 tablespoon whole wheat flour
- 1/2 teaspoon sea salt
- 1/4 teaspoon black pepper
- 8 oz whole wheat fettuccine, cooked

Instructions:

1. Heat the olive oil in a large skillet over medium-high heat.
2. Add the chicken strips and cook for 5-7 minutes, or until cooked through and lightly browned. Remove from the skillet and set aside.
3. In the same skillet, add the garlic and cook for 1-2 minutes until fragrant.
4. Stir in the almond milk, chicken broth, and whole wheat flour. Cook for 2-3 minutes, stirring constantly, until the sauce thickens.
5. Add the Parmesan cheese, sea salt, and black pepper. Stir until the cheese is melted and the sauce is smooth.
6. Return the chicken to the skillet and add the broccoli. Cook for an additional 5 minutes, or until the broccoli is tender.
7. Toss the cooked fettuccine with the chicken and broccoli Alfredo sauce.
8. Serve hot.

Nutrition Info (per serving):

- Calories: 400
- Carbohydrates: 45g
- Protein: 30g
- Fat: 14g
- Fiber: 8g
- Sugar: 3g

Number of Serves: 4
Cooking Time: 30 minutes

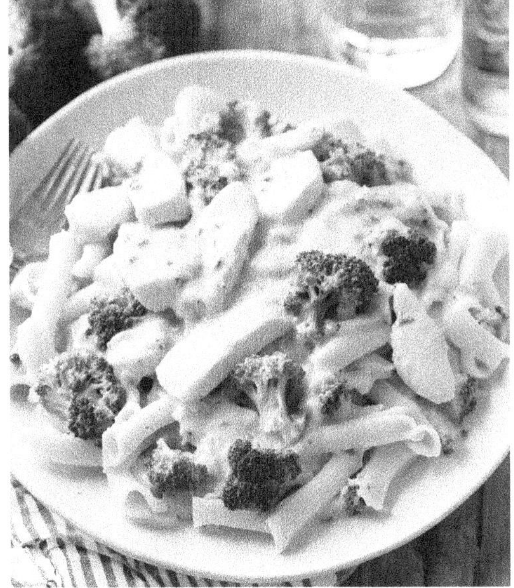

14. Asian Chicken Salad

Ingredients:
- 1 lb boneless, skinless chicken breasts, grilled and sliced
- 4 cups mixed salad greens
- 1 cup shredded red cabbage
- 1 cup shredded carrots
- 1 red bell pepper, thinly sliced
- 1/4 cup fresh cilantro, chopped
- 1/4 cup sliced almonds
- 2 tablespoons sesame seeds
- 2 green onions, sliced

For the Dressing:
- 1/4 cup rice vinegar
- 2 tablespoons soy sauce (low sodium)
- 1 tablespoon sesame oil
- 1 tablespoon honey or maple syrup
- 1 teaspoon grated ginger
- 1 clove garlic, minced

Instructions:
1. In a large bowl, combine the mixed salad greens, shredded red cabbage, shredded carrots, red bell pepper, cilantro, sliced almonds, sesame seeds, and green onions.
2. Add the grilled and sliced chicken to the salad.
3. In a small bowl, whisk together the rice vinegar, soy sauce, sesame oil, honey or maple syrup, grated ginger, and minced garlic.
4. Drizzle the dressing over the salad and toss to combine.
5. Serve immediately.

Nutrition Info (per serving):
- Calories: 350
- Carbohydrates: 18g
- Protein: 30g
- Fat: 20g
- Fiber: 6g
- Sugar: 8g

Number of Serves: 4
Cooking Time: 20 minutes

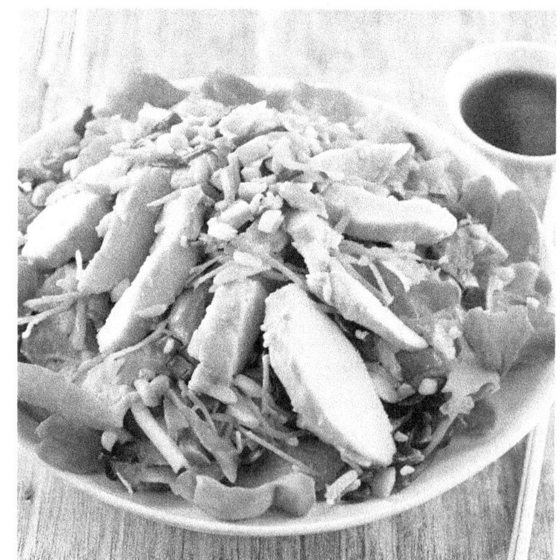

15. Chicken Parmesan

Ingredients:

- 4 boneless, skinless chicken breasts
- 1/2 cup whole wheat bread crumbs
- 1/4 cup grated Parmesan cheese
- 1 teaspoon dried oregano
- 1/2 teaspoon sea salt
- 1/4 teaspoon black pepper
- 1 egg, beaten
- 2 tablespoons olive oil
- 1 cup marinara sauce (low sodium)
- 1 cup shredded mozzarella cheese
- 2 tablespoons fresh basil, chopped

Instructions:

1. Preheat the oven to 375°F (190°C).
2. In a shallow bowl, mix the bread crumbs, Parmesan cheese, dried oregano, sea salt, and black pepper.
3. Dip each chicken breast in the beaten egg, then coat with the bread crumb mixture.
4. Heat the olive oil in a large skillet over medium-high heat. Cook the chicken breasts for 3-4 minutes per side, or until golden brown.
5. Transfer the chicken breasts to a baking dish.
6. Spoon the marinara sauce over the chicken breasts and sprinkle with mozzarella cheese.
7. Bake for 20-25 minutes, or until the chicken is cooked through and the cheese is melted and bubbly.
8. Serve hot, garnished with fresh basil.

Nutrition Info (per serving):

- Calories: 400
- Carbohydrates: 15g
- Protein: 40g
- Fat: 20g
- Fiber: 3g
- Sugar: 4g

Number of Serves: 4
Cooking Time: 30 minutes

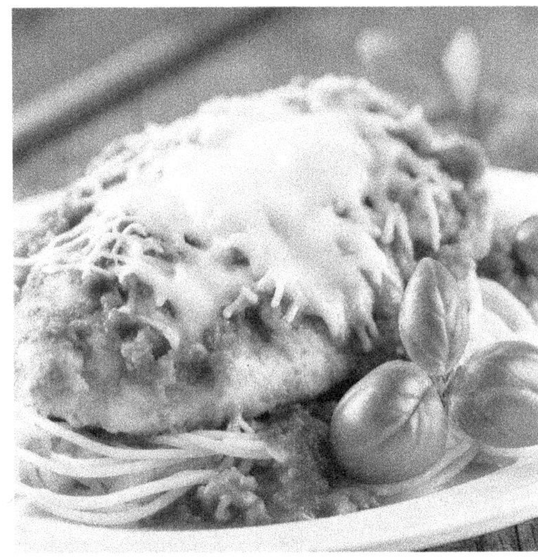

16. Lemon Basil Chicken

Ingredients:

- 4 boneless, skinless chicken breasts
- 2 tablespoons olive oil
- 3 cloves garlic, minced
- 1 lemon, juiced and zested
- 1/4 cup fresh basil, chopped
- 1 teaspoon dried thyme
- 1/2 teaspoon sea salt
- 1/4 teaspoon black pepper

Instructions:

1. In a small bowl, mix the olive oil, garlic, lemon juice, lemon zest, basil, thyme, sea salt, and black pepper.
2. Rub the mixture evenly over the chicken breasts.
3. Preheat the grill to medium-high heat.
4. Grill the chicken breasts for 6-8 minutes per side, or until the internal temperature reaches 165°F (74°C).
5. Serve hot, garnished with additional fresh basil if desired.

Nutrition Info (per serving):

- Calories: 250
- Carbohydrates: 2g
- Protein: 30g
- Fat: 14g
- Fiber: 1g
- Sugar: 1g

Number of Serves: 4

Cooking Time: 20 minutes

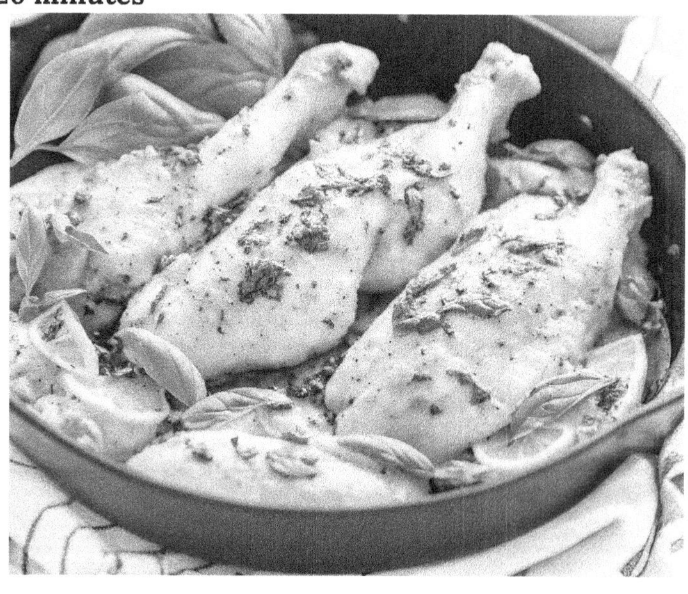

17. Turkey Meatballs in Tomato Basil Sauce

Ingredients:

- 1 lb ground turkey
- 1/2 cup whole wheat bread crumbs
- 1/4 cup grated Parmesan cheese
- 1 egg, beaten
- 2 cloves garlic, minced
- 1 tablespoon fresh parsley, chopped
- 1 teaspoon dried oregano
- 1/2 teaspoon sea salt
- 1/4 teaspoon black pepper
- 2 tablespoons olive oil
- 1 (14 oz) can diced tomatoes
- 1 (14 oz) can tomato sauce (low sodium)
- 1/4 cup fresh basil, chopped

Instructions:

1. In a large bowl, combine the ground turkey, bread crumbs, Parmesan cheese, egg, garlic, parsley, oregano, sea salt, and black pepper. Mix until well combined.
2. Form the mixture into meatballs.
3. Heat the olive oil in a large skillet over medium-high heat. Add the meatballs and cook for 5-7 minutes, turning occasionally, until browned on all sides.
4. Add the diced tomatoes and tomato sauce to the skillet. Bring to a simmer.
5. Reduce heat to low and cook for 15-20 minutes, or until the meatballs are cooked through.
6. Stir in the fresh basil.
7. Serve hot.

Nutrition Info (per serving):

- Calories: 300
- Carbohydrates: 15g
- Protein: 30g
- Fat: 14g
- Fiber: 3g
- Sugar: 6g

Number of Serves: 4

Cooking Time: 30 minutes

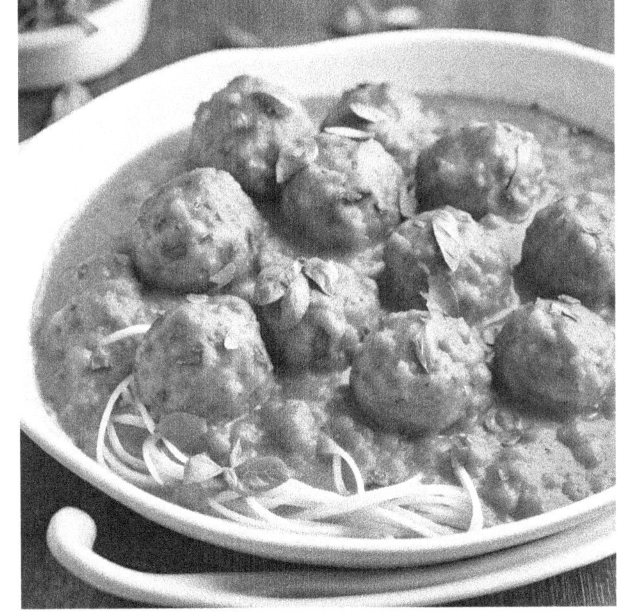

18. Turkey and Vegetable Soup

Ingredients:

- 1 lb ground turkey
- 2 tablespoons olive oil
- 1 large onion, diced
- 3 cloves garlic, minced
- 2 large carrots, diced
- 2 celery stalks, diced
- 1 zucchini, diced
- 1 (14 oz) can diced tomatoes
- 4 cups low sodium chicken broth
- 1 teaspoon dried thyme
- 1/2 teaspoon dried rosemary
- 1/2 teaspoon sea salt
- 1/4 teaspoon black pepper
- 1/4 cup fresh parsley, chopped

Instructions:

1. Heat the olive oil in a large pot over medium heat.
2. Add the ground turkey and cook for 5-7 minutes, or until browned and cooked through. Remove from the pot and set aside.
3. In the same pot, add the onion, garlic, carrots, and celery. Sauté for 5-7 minutes until softened.
4. Stir in the zucchini, diced tomatoes, chicken broth, thyme, rosemary, sea salt, and black pepper. Bring to a simmer.
5. Return the turkey to the pot and cook for 15-20 minutes, or until the vegetables are tender.
6. Stir in the fresh parsley.
7. Serve hot.

Nutrition Info (per serving):

- Calories: 250
- Carbohydrates: 20g
- Protein: 25g
- Fat: 10g
- Fiber: 5g
- Sugar: 8g

Number of Serves: 4

Cooking Time: 35 minutes

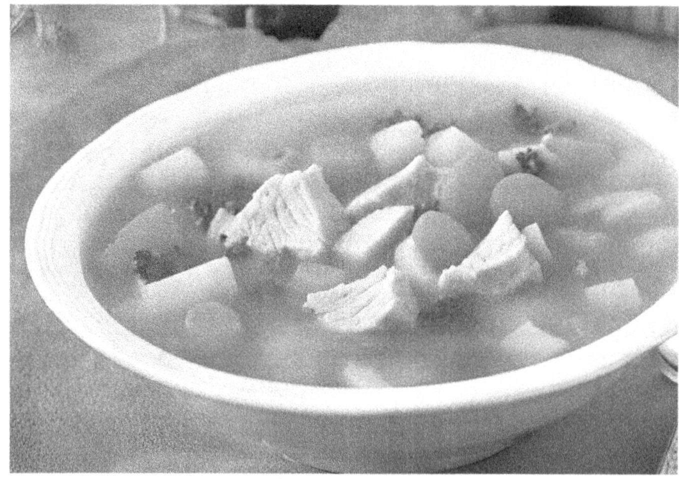

19. Turkey Stir-Fry with Cashews

Ingredients:

- 1 lb ground turkey
- 2 tablespoons olive oil
- 1 red bell pepper, sliced
- 1 yellow bell pepper, sliced
- 1 small onion, sliced
- 2 cloves garlic, minced
- 1 cup snap peas
- 1/4 cup low sodium soy sauce
- 1 tablespoon rice vinegar
- 1 tablespoon honey or maple syrup
- 1/2 teaspoon ground ginger
- 1/4 teaspoon sea salt
- 1/4 teaspoon black pepper
- 1/2 cup unsalted cashews
- 2 green onions, chopped (for garnish)

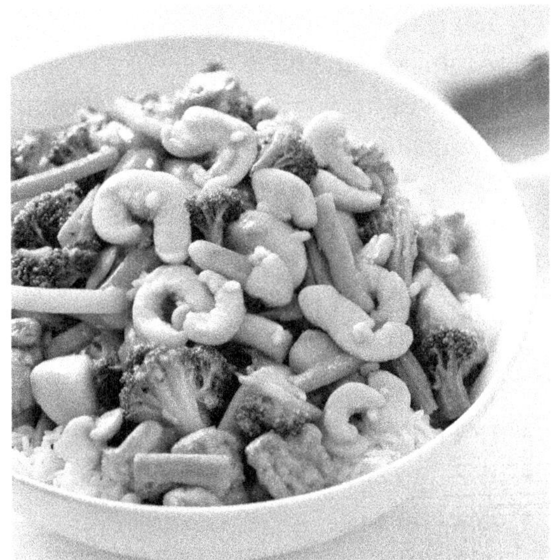

Instructions:

1. Heat 1 tablespoon of olive oil in a large skillet or wok over medium-high heat.
2. Add the ground turkey and cook for 5-7 minutes until browned and cooked through. Remove from the skillet and set aside.
3. In the same skillet, heat the remaining olive oil.
4. Add the red bell pepper, yellow bell pepper, and onion. Stir-fry for 3-4 minutes until tender.
5. Add the garlic and snap peas, stir-frying for an additional 2 minutes.
6. Return the cooked turkey to the skillet.
7. In a small bowl, mix the soy sauce, rice vinegar, honey or maple syrup, ground ginger, sea salt, and black pepper. Pour over the turkey and vegetables.
8. Stir in the cashews and cook for another 2-3 minutes until heated through.
9. Serve hot, garnished with chopped green onions.

Nutrition Info (per serving):

- Calories: 350
- Carbohydrates: 20g
- Protein: 30g
- Fat: 18g
- Fiber: 4g
- Sugar: 6g

Number of Serves: 4
Cooking Time: 20 minutes

20. Turkey Taco Salad

Ingredients:

- 1 lb ground turkey
- 2 tablespoons olive oil
- 1 packet taco seasoning (low sodium)
- 4 cups mixed salad greens
- 1 cup cherry tomatoes, halved
- 1 cup corn kernels (fresh or frozen)
- 1/2 cup black beans, rinsed and drained
- 1/2 red onion, diced
- 1 avocado, diced
- 1/4 cup fresh cilantro, chopped
- 1/4 cup shredded cheddar cheese (optional)
- 1/2 cup Greek yogurt (unsweetened)
- 1/4 cup salsa

Instructions:

1. Heat the olive oil in a large skillet over medium-high heat.
2. Add the ground turkey and cook for 5-7 minutes until browned and cooked through.
3. Stir in the taco seasoning and cook for another 2-3 minutes until well combined. Remove from heat.
4. In a large bowl, combine the mixed salad greens, cherry tomatoes, corn kernels, black beans, red onion, avocado, and cilantro.
5. Top the salad with the cooked turkey mixture.
6. Sprinkle with shredded cheddar cheese, if using.
7. In a small bowl, mix the Greek yogurt and salsa to make the dressing.
8. Drizzle the dressing over the salad and serve immediately.

Nutrition Info (per serving):

- Calories: 400
- Carbohydrates: 30g
- Protein: 30g
- Fat: 18g
- Fiber: 8g
- Sugar: 6g

Number of Serves: 4

Cooking Time: 20 minutes

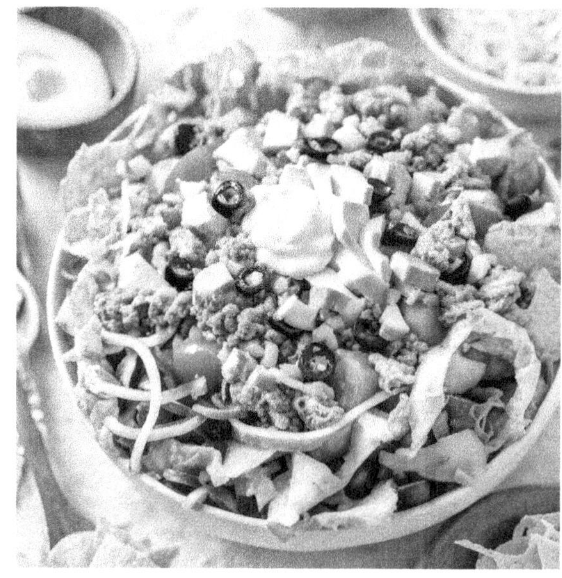

21. Baked Turkey and Spinach Meatballs

Ingredients:

- 1 lb ground turkey
- 1 cup fresh spinach, finely chopped
- 1/2 cup whole wheat bread crumbs
- 1/4 cup grated Parmesan cheese
- 1 egg, beaten
- 2 cloves garlic, minced
- 1 teaspoon dried oregano
- 1/2 teaspoon sea salt
- 1/4 teaspoon black pepper
- 1 tablespoon olive oil (for greasing baking sheet)

Instructions:

1. Preheat the oven to 375°F (190°C). Grease a baking sheet with olive oil.
2. In a large bowl, combine the ground turkey, spinach, bread crumbs, Parmesan cheese, egg, garlic, oregano, sea salt, and black pepper. Mix until well combined.
3. Form the mixture into meatballs and place them on the prepared baking sheet.
4. Bake for 20-25 minutes, or until the meatballs are cooked through and golden brown.
5. Serve hot.

Nutrition Info (per serving):

- Calories: 250
- Carbohydrates: 10g
- Protein: 30g
- Fat: 10g
- Fiber: 2g
- Sugar: 1g

Number of Serves: 4
Cooking Time: 25 minutes

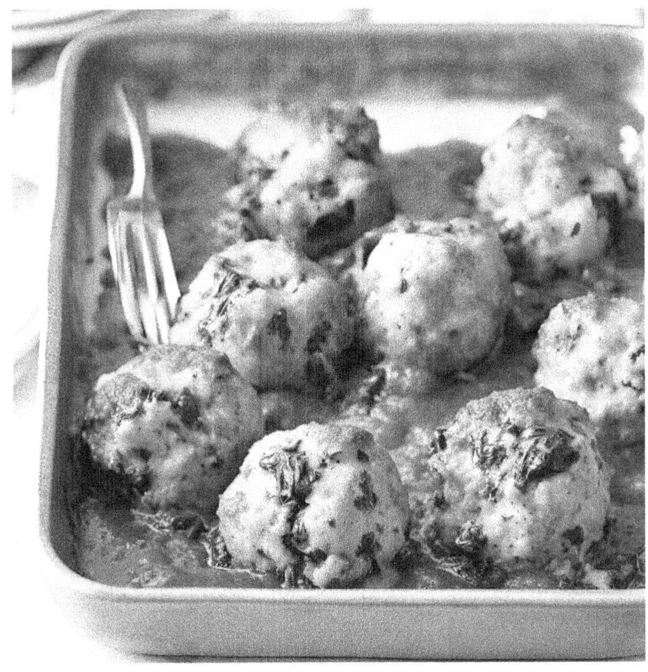

22. Smoked Turkey Breast

Ingredients:

- 4 lb turkey breast
- 2 tablespoons olive oil
- 1 tablespoon smoked paprika
- 1 teaspoon garlic powder
- 1 teaspoon onion powder
- 1 teaspoon dried thyme
- 1/2 teaspoon sea salt
- 1/4 teaspoon black pepper
- 1/4 cup apple cider vinegar

Instructions:

1. Preheat the smoker to 225°F (107°C).
2. In a small bowl, mix the olive oil, smoked paprika, garlic powder, onion powder, thyme, sea salt, and black pepper.
3. Rub the mixture all over the turkey breast.
4. Place the turkey breast in the smoker.
5. Smoke the turkey for 3-4 hours, or until the internal temperature reaches 165°F (74°C).
6. Brush the turkey breast with apple cider vinegar every hour to keep it moist.
7. Let the turkey rest for 10 minutes before slicing.
8. Serve hot.

Nutrition Info (per serving):

- Calories: 300
- Carbohydrates: 2g
- Protein: 45g
- Fat: 12g
- Fiber: 0g
- Sugar: 1g

Number of Serves: 8
Cooking Time: 4 hours

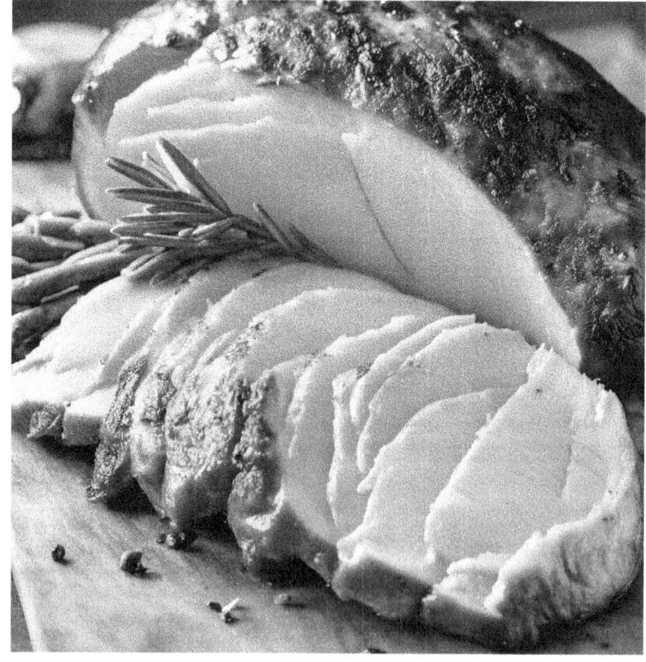

23. Duck Breast with Orange Sauce

Ingredients:

- 4 duck breasts
- 1/2 teaspoon sea salt
- 1/4 teaspoon black pepper
- 1/2 cup orange juice
- 1/4 cup chicken broth (low sodium)
- 1 tablespoon honey or maple syrup
- 1 tablespoon balsamic vinegar
- 1 teaspoon orange zest
- 1 tablespoon fresh thyme, chopped

Instructions:

1. Preheat the oven to 400°F (200°C).
2. Score the skin of the duck breasts in a crosshatch pattern. Season with sea salt and black pepper.
3. Place the duck breasts, skin-side down, in a cold oven-safe skillet. Cook over medium heat for 6-8 minutes until the skin is crispy and browned. Flip the duck breasts and cook for another 2 minutes.
4. Transfer the skillet to the oven and bake for 5-7 minutes, or until the internal temperature reaches 135°F (57°C) for medium-rare.
5. Remove the duck breasts from the skillet and let rest.
6. In the same skillet, add the orange juice, chicken broth, honey or maple syrup, balsamic vinegar, and orange zest. Cook over medium heat for 5 minutes until the sauce has reduced and thickened.
7. Stir in the fresh thyme.
8. Serve the duck breasts sliced, with the orange sauce drizzled on top.

Nutrition Info (per serving):

- Calories: 400
- Carbohydrates: 10g
- Protein: 30g
- Fat: 26g
- Fiber: 0g
- Sugar: 8g

Number of Serves: 4
Cooking Time: 25 minutes

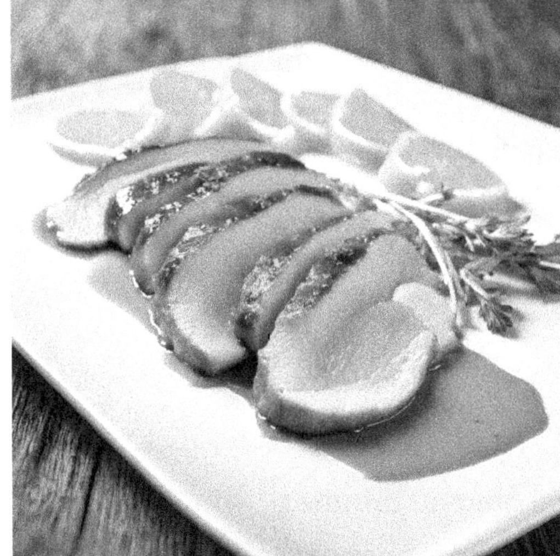

24. Cornish Hen with Wild Rice Stuffing

Ingredients:

- 2 Cornish hens
- 2 tablespoons olive oil
- 1 teaspoon sea salt
- 1/2 teaspoon black pepper
- 1 teaspoon dried thyme
- 1 cup wild rice
- 2 cups low sodium chicken broth
- 1 small onion, diced
- 2 cloves garlic, minced
- 1/2 cup dried cranberries
- 1/2 cup chopped pecans
- 1/4 cup fresh parsley, chopped

Instructions:

1. Preheat the oven to 375°F (190°C).
2. Rinse the wild rice under cold water. In a medium saucepan, bring the chicken broth to a boil. Add the wild rice, reduce heat, cover, and simmer for 45 minutes, or until the rice is tender and the liquid is absorbed.
3. In a skillet, heat 1 tablespoon of olive oil over medium heat. Add the onion and garlic, sautéing for 3-4 minutes until softened.
4. Stir in the cooked wild rice, dried cranberries, chopped pecans, and fresh parsley.
5. Rinse and pat dry the Cornish hens. Rub the remaining olive oil, sea salt, black pepper, and dried thyme all over the hens.
6. Stuff the hens with the wild rice mixture.
7. Place the hens in a roasting pan and roast for 50-60 minutes, or until the internal temperature reaches 165°F (74°C).
8. Let the hens rest for 10 minutes before serving.
9. Serve hot.

Nutrition Info (per serving):

- Calories: 500
- Carbohydrates: 30g
- Protein: 40g
- Fat: 26g
- Fiber: 4g
- Sugar: 8g

Number of Serves: 4

Cooking Time: 1 hour 10 minutes

25. Guinea Fowl with Lemon and Thyme

Ingredients:

- 1 whole guinea fowl (about 3 lbs)
- 2 tablespoons olive oil
- 2 lemons, sliced
- 4 cloves garlic, minced
- 1 tablespoon fresh thyme leaves
- 1 teaspoon sea salt
- 1/2 teaspoon black pepper

Instructions:

1. Preheat the oven to 375°F (190°C).
2. Rub the guinea fowl with olive oil, garlic, thyme, sea salt, and black pepper.
3. Place the lemon slices inside the cavity and on top of the guinea fowl.
4. Place the guinea fowl in a roasting pan and roast for 1 1/2 hours, or until the internal temperature reaches 165°F (74°C).
5. Let the guinea fowl rest for 10 minutes before carving.
6. Serve hot.

Nutrition Info (per serving):

- Calories: 400
- Carbohydrates: 4g
- Protein: 32g
- Fat: 28g
- Fiber: 1g
- Sugar: 1g

Number of Serves: 4
Cooking Time: 1 hour 40 minutes

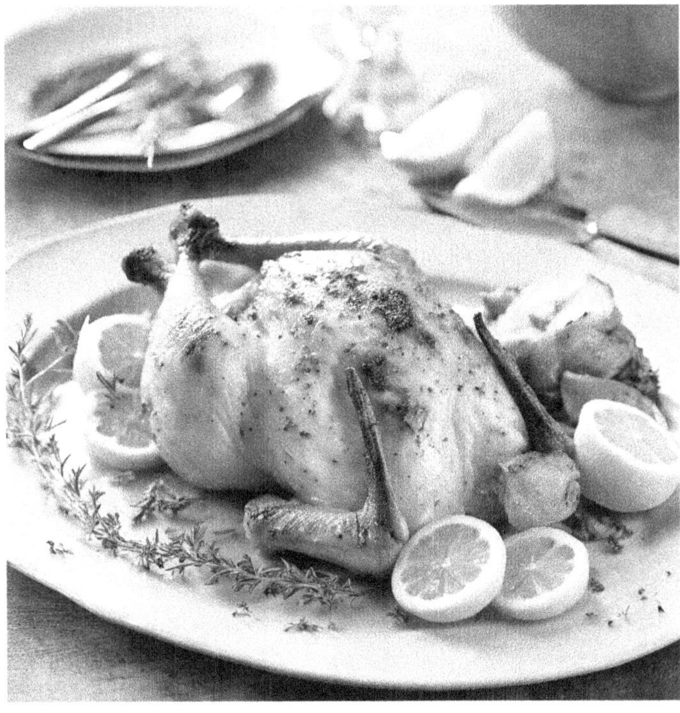

v26. Grilled Pigeon with Mediterranean Vegetables

Ingredients:

- 4 pigeons, cleaned
- 2 tablespoons olive oil
- 2 cloves garlic, minced
- 1 tablespoon fresh oregano, chopped
- 1 teaspoon sea salt
- 1/2 teaspoon black pepper
- 2 zucchini, sliced
- 2 red bell peppers, sliced
- 1 large red onion, sliced
- 1 lemon, juiced

Instructions:

1. Preheat the grill to medium-high heat.
2. In a small bowl, mix the olive oil, garlic, oregano, sea salt, and black pepper.
3. Rub the mixture over the pigeons and let marinate for 15 minutes.
4. Grill the pigeons for 6-8 minutes per side, or until the internal temperature reaches 165°F (74°C).
5. While the pigeons are grilling, toss the zucchini, red bell peppers, and red onion with lemon juice and a little olive oil.
6. Grill the vegetables for 4-5 minutes per side, until tender and slightly charred.
7. Serve the grilled pigeons with the Mediterranean vegetables.

Nutrition Info (per serving):

- Calories: 450
- Carbohydrates: 10g
- Protein: 38g
- Fat: 28g
- Fiber: 4g
- Sugar: 5g

Number of Serves: 4

Cooking Time: 25 minutes

27. Braised Rabbit with Garlic and Rosemary

Ingredients:

- 1 whole rabbit (about 2-3 lbs), cut into pieces
- 2 tablespoons olive oil
- 1 large onion, diced
- 4 cloves garlic, minced
- 1 tablespoon fresh rosemary, chopped
- 1 cup dry white wine
- 2 cups low sodium chicken broth
- 1 teaspoon sea salt
- 1/2 teaspoon black pepper
- 2 large carrots, sliced
- 2 celery stalks, sliced

Instructions:

1. Preheat the oven to 350°F (175°C).
2. In a large oven-safe pot, heat the olive oil over medium-high heat.
3. Add the rabbit pieces and brown on all sides, about 5-7 minutes. Remove and set aside.
4. In the same pot, add the onion, garlic, and rosemary. Sauté for 3-4 minutes until softened.
5. Stir in the white wine and cook for 2-3 minutes until reduced by half.
6. Add the chicken broth, sea salt, and black pepper. Return the rabbit to the pot and add the carrots and celery.
7. Cover and braise in the oven for 1 1/2 hours, or until the rabbit is tender.
8. Serve hot.

Nutrition Info (per serving):

- Calories: 400
- Carbohydrates: 10g
- Protein: 35g
- Fat: 20g
- Fiber: 3g
- Sugar: 5g

Number of Serves: 4

Cooking Time: 1 hour 45 minutes

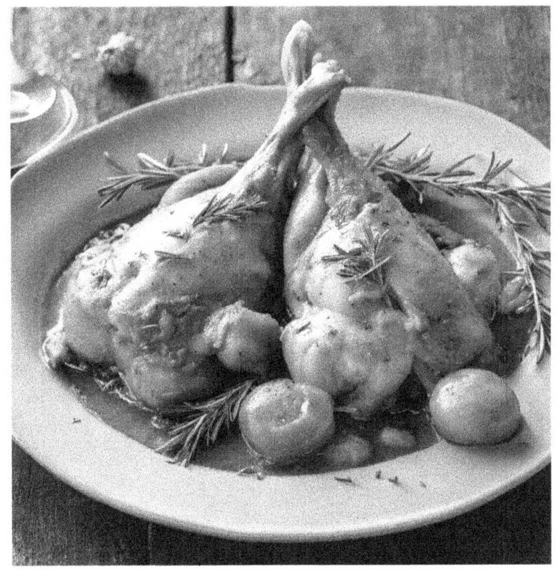

28. Game Hen Stew with Barley

Ingredients:

- 2 game hens, cut into pieces
- 2 tablespoons olive oil
- 1 large onion, diced
- 3 cloves garlic, minced
- 2 large carrots, sliced
- 2 celery stalks, sliced
- 1 cup pearl barley
- 4 cups low sodium chicken broth
- 1 teaspoon dried thyme
- 1/2 teaspoon sea salt
- 1/4 teaspoon black pepper
- 1/4 cup fresh parsley, chopped

Instructions:

1. In a large pot, heat the olive oil over medium-high heat.
2. Add the game hen pieces and brown on all sides, about 5-7 minutes. Remove and set aside.
3. In the same pot, add the onion, garlic, carrots, and celery. Sauté for 5-7 minutes until softened.
4. Stir in the pearl barley, chicken broth, thyme, sea salt, and black pepper. Bring to a simmer.
5. Return the game hen pieces to the pot.
6. Cover and cook for 1 hour, or until the barley is tender and the game hen is cooked through.
7. Stir in the fresh parsley before serving.
8. Serve hot.

Nutrition Info (per serving):

- Calories: 450
- Carbohydrates: 30g
- Protein: 32g
- Fat: 20g
- Fiber: 8g
- Sugar: 6g

Number of Serves: 4

Cooking Time: 1 hour 20 minutes

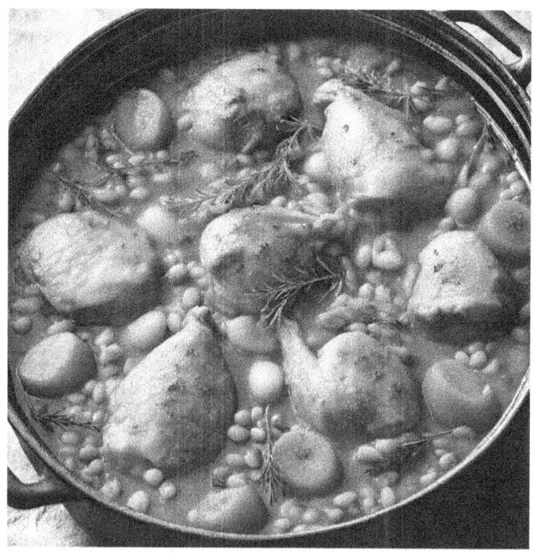

29. Roasted Partridge with Pear

Ingredients:

- 4 partridges
- 2 tablespoons olive oil
- 2 cloves garlic, minced
- 1 teaspoon dried thyme
- 1/2 teaspoon sea salt
- 1/4 teaspoon black pepper
- 2 pears, halved and cored
- 1/4 cup dry white wine

Instructions:

1. Preheat the oven to 375°F (190°C).
2. In a small bowl, mix the olive oil, garlic, thyme, sea salt, and black pepper.
3. Rub the mixture over the partridges.
4. Place the partridges in a roasting pan and arrange the pear halves around them.
5. Pour the white wine over the partridges and pears.
6. Roast for 45-50 minutes, or until the partridges are cooked through and the internal temperature reaches 165°F (74°C).
7. Let the partridges rest for 10 minutes before serving.
8. Serve hot with the roasted pears.

Nutrition Info (per serving):

- Calories: 400
- Carbohydrates: 15g
- Protein: 32g
- Fat: 22g
- Fiber: 3g
- Sugar: 10g

Number of Serves: 4
Cooking Time: 50 minutes

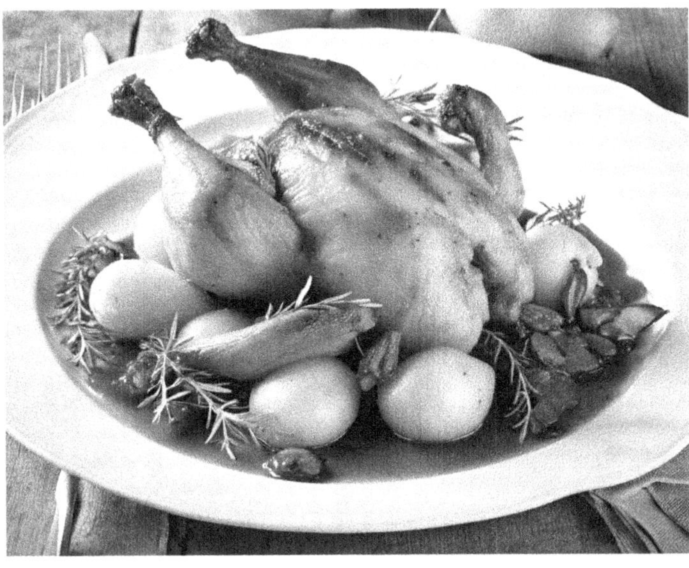

30. Smoked Duck Salad with Pomegranate

Ingredients:

- 1 smoked duck breast
- 4 cups mixed salad greens
- 1/2 cup pomegranate seeds
- 1/4 cup walnuts, toasted
- 1/4 cup crumbled feta cheese
- 1/4 cup olive oil
- 2 tablespoons balsamic vinegar
- 1 tablespoon honey or maple syrup
- 1 teaspoon Dijon mustard
- 1/4 teaspoon sea salt
- 1/4 teaspoon black pepper

Instructions:

1. Thinly slice the smoked duck breast.
2. In a large bowl, combine the salad greens, pomegranate seeds, toasted walnuts, and crumbled feta cheese.
3. In a small bowl, whisk together the olive oil, balsamic vinegar, honey or maple syrup, Dijon mustard, sea salt, and black pepper.
4. Drizzle the dressing over the salad and toss to combine.
5. Arrange the sliced smoked duck breast on top of the salad.
6. Serve immediately.

Nutrition Info (per serving):

- Calories: 350
- Carbohydrates: 12g
- Protein: 20g
- Fat: 24g
- Fiber: 4g
- Sugar: 8g

Number of Serves: 4
Cooking Time: 15 minutes

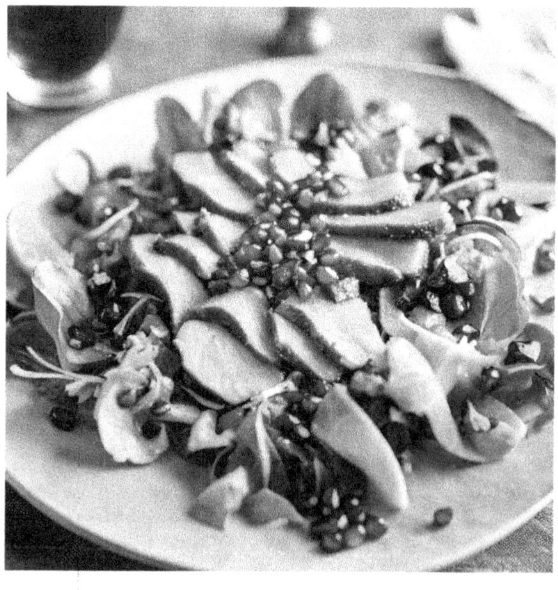

Soup & Stew Recipes

1. Brazilian Black Bean Stew (Feijoada)

Ingredients:

- 1 lb dried black beans, rinsed and soaked overnight
- 1 lb lean pork shoulder, cubed
- 1/2 lb turkey sausage, sliced
- 1 large onion, diced
- 4 cloves garlic, minced
- 2 tablespoons olive oil
- 1 bay leaf
- 1 teaspoon cumin
- 1 teaspoon smoked paprika
- 1/2 teaspoon sea salt
- 1/4 teaspoon black pepper
- 4 cups low sodium chicken broth
- 2 cups water
- 1 orange, sliced (for garnish)
- Fresh cilantro, chopped (for garnish)

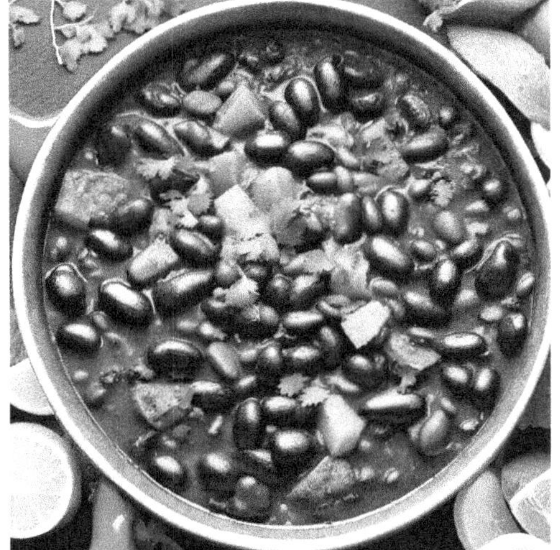

Instructions:

1. Drain and rinse the soaked black beans.
2. In a large pot, heat the olive oil over medium-high heat.
3. Add the pork shoulder and turkey sausage, browning on all sides, about 5-7 minutes.
4. Add the onion and garlic, sautéing for 3-4 minutes until softened.
5. Stir in the black beans, bay leaf, cumin, smoked paprika, sea salt, and black pepper.
6. Pour in the chicken broth and water, bringing to a boil.
7. Reduce heat to low, cover, and simmer for 1 1/2 to 2 hours, or until the beans and meat are tender.
8. Remove the bay leaf before serving.
9. Serve hot, garnished with orange slices and fresh cilantro.

Nutrition Info (per serving):

- Calories: 350
- Carbohydrates: 30g
- Protein: 28g
- Fat: 12g
- Fiber: 12g
- Sugar: 2g

Number of Serves: 6

Cooking Time: 2 hours 15 minutes

2. White Bean and Kale Stew

Ingredients:

- 1 lb dried white beans, rinsed and soaked overnight
- 1 large onion, diced
- 3 cloves garlic, minced
- 2 tablespoons olive oil
- 1 large carrot, diced
- 2 celery stalks, diced
- 4 cups low sodium vegetable broth
- 2 cups water
- 1 teaspoon dried thyme
- 1/2 teaspoon dried rosemary
- 1/2 teaspoon sea salt
- 1/4 teaspoon black pepper
- 4 cups chopped kale
- 1/4 cup fresh parsley, chopped

Instructions:

1. Drain and rinse the soaked white beans.
2. In a large pot, heat the olive oil over medium heat.
3. Add the onion, garlic, carrot, and celery, sautéing for 5-7 minutes until softened.
4. Stir in the white beans, vegetable broth, water, thyme, rosemary, sea salt, and black pepper.
5. Bring to a boil, then reduce heat to low, cover, and simmer for 1 1/2 to 2 hours, or until the beans are tender.
6. Stir in the chopped kale and cook for an additional 10 minutes.
7. Serve hot, garnished with fresh parsley.

Nutrition Info (per serving):

- Calories: 300
- Carbohydrates: 45g
- Protein: 15g
- Fat: 8g
- Fiber: 15g
- Sugar: 6g

Number of Serves: 6

Cooking Time: 2 hours 15 minutes

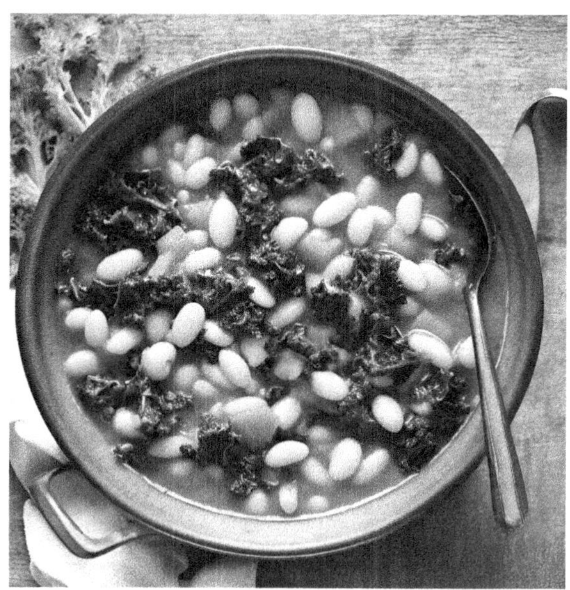

3. Fisherman's Stew

Ingredients:

- 1 lb firm white fish (such as cod or halibut), cut into chunks
- 1/2 lb shrimp, peeled and deveined
- 1/2 lb mussels, cleaned
- 1 large onion, diced
- 3 cloves garlic, minced
- 2 tablespoons olive oil
- 1 (14 oz) can diced tomatoes
- 4 cups low sodium fish broth
- 1 cup dry white wine
- 1 teaspoon dried thyme
- 1 teaspoon smoked paprika
- 1/2 teaspoon sea salt
- 1/4 teaspoon black pepper
- 1/4 cup fresh parsley, chopped

Instructions:

1. In a large pot, heat the olive oil over medium heat.
2. Add the onion and garlic, sautéing for 3-4 minutes until softened.
3. Stir in the diced tomatoes, fish broth, white wine, thyme, smoked paprika, sea salt, and black pepper. Bring to a simmer.
4. Add the fish chunks and shrimp, cooking for 5-7 minutes until the fish is opaque and the shrimp are pink.
5. Add the mussels and cook for another 5 minutes, or until the mussels open. Discard any that do not open.
6. Serve hot, garnished with fresh parsley.

Nutrition Info (per serving):

- Calories: 350
- Carbohydrates: 12g
- Protein: 35g
- Fat: 12g
- Fiber: 2g
- Sugar: 4g

Number of Serves: 6

Cooking Time: 25 minutes

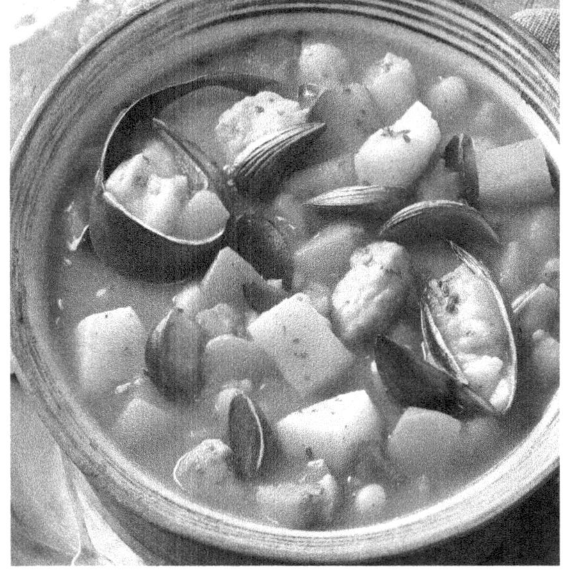

4. Moroccan Lamb Stew

Ingredients:

- 1 1/2 lbs lamb shoulder, cut into chunks
- 2 tablespoons olive oil
- 1 large onion, diced
- 3 cloves garlic, minced
- 2 large carrots, sliced
- 2 celery stalks, sliced
- 1 (14 oz) can diced tomatoes
- 4 cups low sodium beef broth
- 1 teaspoon ground cumin
- 1 teaspoon ground coriander
- 1 teaspoon ground cinnamon
- 1/2 teaspoon ground turmeric
- 1/2 teaspoon sea salt
- 1/4 teaspoon black pepper
- 1/2 cup dried apricots, chopped
- 1/4 cup fresh cilantro, chopped

Instructions:

1. In a large pot, heat the olive oil over medium-high heat.
2. Add the lamb chunks and brown on all sides, about 5-7 minutes. Remove and set aside.
3. In the same pot, add the onion, garlic, carrots, and celery. Sauté for 5-7 minutes until softened.
4. Stir in the diced tomatoes, beef broth, cumin, coriander, cinnamon, turmeric, sea salt, and black pepper. Bring to a simmer.
5. Return the lamb to the pot and add the dried apricots.
6. Cover and simmer for 1 1/2 to 2 hours, or until the lamb is tender.
7. Serve hot, garnished with fresh cilantro.

Nutrition Info (per serving):

- Calories: 400
- Carbohydrates: 25g
- Protein: 30g
- Fat: 20g
- Fiber: 5g
- Sugar: 10g

Number of Serves: 6

Cooking Time: 2 hours 15 minutes

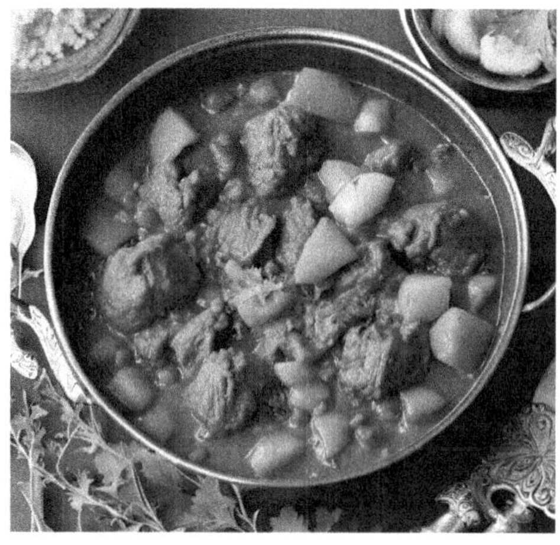

5. Split Pea Soup

Ingredients:

- 1 lb dried split peas, rinsed
- 1 large onion, diced
- 3 cloves garlic, minced
- 2 tablespoons olive oil
- 2 large carrots, diced
- 2 celery stalks, diced
- 6 cups low sodium vegetable broth
- 2 cups water
- 1 bay leaf
- 1 teaspoon dried thyme
- 1/2 teaspoon sea salt
- 1/4 teaspoon black pepper
- 1/4 cup fresh parsley, chopped

Instructions:

1. In a large pot, heat the olive oil over medium heat.
2. Add the onion, garlic, carrots, and celery. Sauté for 5-7 minutes until softened.
3. Stir in the split peas, vegetable broth, water, bay leaf, thyme, sea salt, and black pepper. Bring to a boil.
4. Reduce heat to low, cover, and simmer for 1 1/2 hours, or until the peas are tender.
5. Remove the bay leaf before serving.
6. Serve hot, garnished with fresh parsley.

Nutrition Info (per serving):

- Calories: 300
- Carbohydrates: 50g
- Protein: 18g
- Fat: 6g
- Fiber: 20g
- Sugar: 8g

Number of Serves: 6
Cooking Time: 1 hour 45 minutes

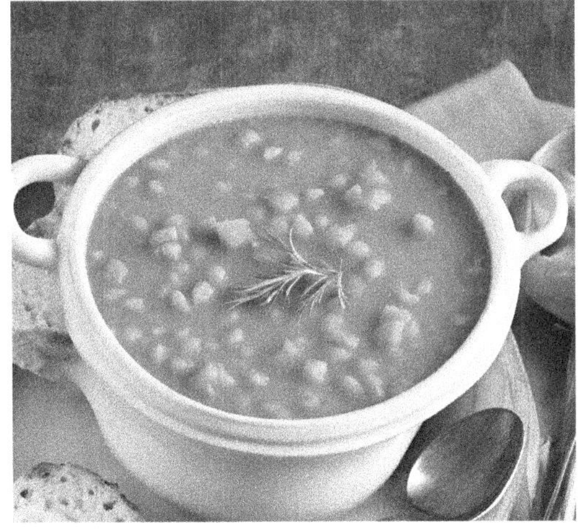

6. Miso Soup with Tofu and Seaweed

Ingredients:

- 6 cups water
- 1/4 cup miso paste
- 1 cup silken tofu, cubed
- 1/4 cup dried seaweed (wakame), soaked and drained
- 2 green onions, sliced
- 1 tablespoon soy sauce (low sodium)

Instructions:

1. In a large pot, bring the water to a simmer.
2. Whisk in the miso paste until fully dissolved.
3. Add the tofu cubes and soaked seaweed. Cook for 5 minutes.
4. Stir in the soy sauce and green onions.
5. Serve hot.

Nutrition Info (per serving):

- Calories: 100
- Carbohydrates: 8g
- Protein: 7g
- Fat: 4g
- Fiber: 2g
- Sugar: 2g

Number of Serves: 4
Cooking Time: 15 minutes

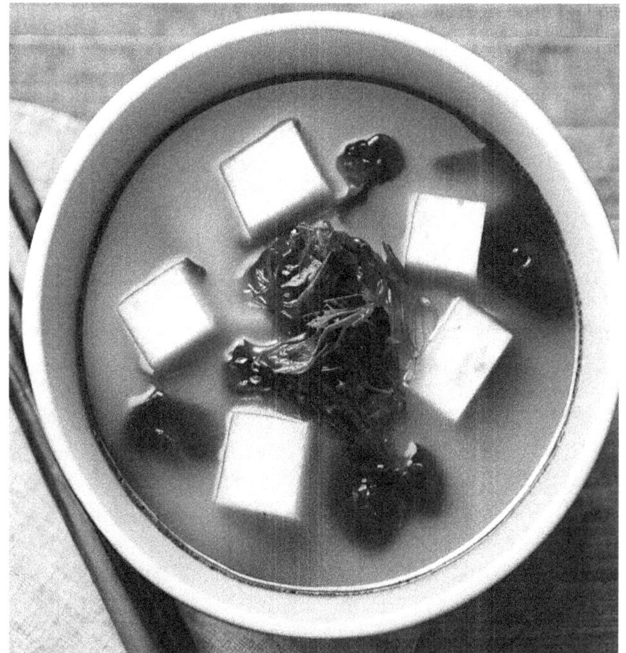

7. Minestrone Soup

Ingredients:

- 2 tablespoons olive oil
- 1 large onion, diced
- 3 cloves garlic, minced
- 2 large carrots, diced
- 2 celery stalks, diced
- 1 zucchini, diced
- 1 (14 oz) can diced tomatoes
- 4 cups low sodium vegetable broth
- 2 cups water
- 1 cup cooked kidney beans
- 1 cup cooked cannellini beans
- 1 teaspoon dried oregano
- 1 teaspoon dried basil
- 1/2 teaspoon sea salt
- 1/4 teaspoon black pepper
- 1 cup whole wheat pasta, cooked
- 1/4 cup fresh parsley, chopped

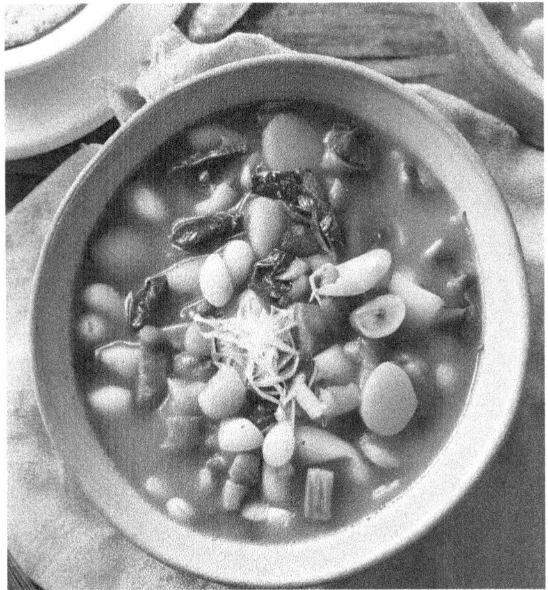

Instructions:

1. In a large pot, heat the olive oil over medium heat.
2. Add the onion, garlic, carrots, celery, and zucchini. Sauté for 5-7 minutes until softened.
3. Stir in the diced tomatoes, vegetable broth, water, kidney beans, cannellini beans, oregano, basil, sea salt, and black pepper. Bring to a simmer.
4. Cook for 20-25 minutes, or until the vegetables are tender.
5. Stir in the cooked pasta and cook for an additional 5 minutes.
6. Serve hot, garnished with fresh parsley.

Nutrition Info (per serving):

- Calories: 300
- Carbohydrates: 50g
- Protein: 12g
- Fat: 8g
- Fiber: 10g
- Sugar: 10g

Number of Serves: 6
Cooking Time: 35 minutes

8. Potato Leek Soup

Ingredients:

- 2 tablespoons olive oil
- 3 leeks, cleaned and sliced
- 2 cloves garlic, minced
- 4 large potatoes, peeled and diced
- 6 cups low sodium vegetable broth
- 1 cup unsweetened almond milk
- 1 teaspoon dried thyme
- 1/2 teaspoon sea salt
- 1/4 teaspoon black pepper
- 1/4 cup fresh chives, chopped (for garnish)

Instructions:

1. In a large pot, heat the olive oil over medium heat.
2. Add the leeks and garlic, sautéing for 5-7 minutes until softened.
3. Stir in the potatoes, vegetable broth, almond milk, thyme, sea salt, and black pepper. Bring to a boil.
4. Reduce heat to low, cover, and simmer for 20-25 minutes, or until the potatoes are tender.
5. Using an immersion blender, blend the soup until smooth.
6. Serve hot, garnished with fresh chives.

Nutrition Info (per serving):

- Calories: 250
- Carbohydrates: 45g
- Protein: 5g
- Fat: 8g
- Fiber: 6g
- Sugar: 6g

Number of Serves: 6
Cooking Time: 35 minutes

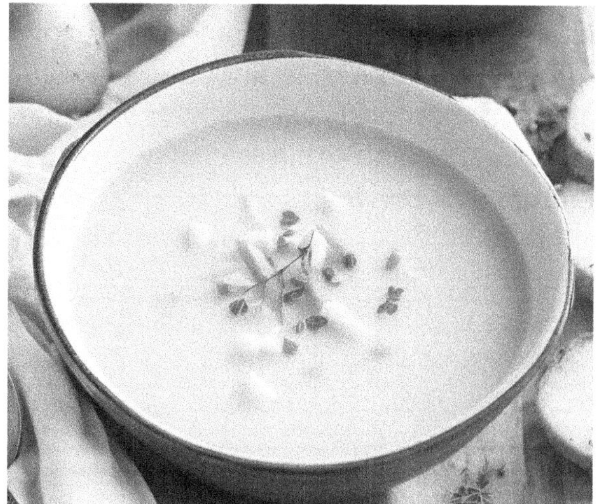

10-WEEK MEAL PLAN

Week 1
Day 1:
- Breakfast: Blueberry and Lemon Oatmeal
- Lunch: White Bean and Kale Stew
- Dinner: Grilled Chicken Breast with Herbed Quinoa

Day 2:
- Breakfast: Cauliflower Breakfast Skillet
- Lunch: Miso Soup with Tofu and Seaweed
- Dinner: Brazilian Black Bean Stew (Feijoada)

Day 3:
- Breakfast: Hummus and Vegetable Breakfast Bowl
- Lunch: Chicken and Broccoli Alfredo
- Dinner: Moroccan Lamb Stew

Day 4:
- Breakfast: Overnight Oats with Chia and Flaxseeds
- Lunch: Fisherman's Stew
- Dinner: Lemon Basil Chicken

Day 5:
- Breakfast: Soy Yogurt with Mixed Berries
- Lunch: Chicken Taco Salad
- Dinner: Baked Lemon Sole with Parmesan

Day 6:
- Breakfast: Cranberry Almond Breakfast Cookies
- Lunch: Minestrone Soup
- Dinner: Moroccan Chicken Tagine

Day 7:
- Breakfast: Spiced Lentil and Rice Porridge
- Lunch: Turkey Stir-Fry with Cashews
- Dinner: Roasted Partridge with Pear

Week 2
Day 1:
- Breakfast: Maple Glazed Carrot Muffins
- Lunch: Chicken and Vegetable Stir-Fry
- Dinner: Split Pea Soup

Day 2:
- Breakfast: Vegetable and Goat Cheese Frittata
- Lunch: Asian Chicken Salad
- Dinner: Classic Beef Stew

Day 3:
- Breakfast: Mango and Lime Quinoa Salad
- Lunch: Thai Chicken Coconut Curry
- Dinner: Grilled Salmon with Lemon and Herbs

Day 4:
- Breakfast: Protein-Packed Breakfast Bars
- Lunch: Smoked Duck Salad with Pomegranate
- Dinner: Lamb and Spinach Lasagna

Day 5:
- Breakfast: Almond Butter and Banana Sandwich
- Lunch: Chicken Piccata with Capers
- Dinner: Seafood Paella

Day 6:
- Breakfast: Kale and Potato Breakfast Hash
- Lunch: Beef and Barley Soup
- Dinner: Game Hen Stew with Barley

Day 7:
- Breakfast: Buckwheat Pancakes
- Lunch: Turkey and Vegetable Soup
- Dinner: Duck Breast with Orange Sauce

Week 3

Day 1:
- Breakfast: Raspberry Almond Muffins
- Lunch: Grilled Beef Skewers
- Dinner: Potato Leek Soup

Day 2:
- Breakfast: Tofu Scramble
- Lunch: Grilled Pigeon with Mediterranean Vegetables
- Dinner: Baked Turkey and Spinach Meatballs

Day 3:
- Breakfast: Baked Pears with Walnuts and Honey
- Lunch: Chicken Paella
- Dinner: Roasted Partridge with Pear

Day 4:
- Breakfast: Pumpkin Spice Smoothie
- Lunch: Grilled Octopus with Olives and Oregano
- Dinner: Turkey Stir-Fry with Cashews

Day 5:
- Breakfast: Quinoa Porridge
- Lunch: Spicy Tuna Poke Bowl
- Dinner: Moroccan Chicken Tagine

Day 6:
- Breakfast: Spinach and Feta Omelette
- Lunch: Buffalo Chicken Wrap
- Dinner: Slow Cooker Pot Roast

Day 7:
- Breakfast: Chicken Sausage and Sweet Potato Hash
- Lunch: Minestrone Soup
- Dinner: Balsamic Glazed Beef Roast

Week 4

Day 1:
- Breakfast: Salted Peanut Butter Oatmeal
- Lunch: White Bean and Kale Stew
- Dinner: Cornish Hen with Wild Rice Stuffing

Day 2:
- Breakfast: Egg Muffins
- Lunch: Mediterranean Lamb Meatballs
- Dinner: Turkey Meatballs in Tomato Basil Sauce

Day 3:
- Breakfast: Greek Yogurt Parfait
- Lunch: Grilled Beef Skewers
- Dinner: Beef Gyros

Day 4:
- Breakfast: Banana Oatmeal Pancakes
- Lunch: Turkey Taco Salad
- Dinner: Braised Rabbit with Garlic and Rosemary

Day 5:
- Breakfast: Overnight Oats with Chia and Flaxseeds
- Lunch: Shrimp Scampi with Zucchini Noodles
- Dinner: Chicken Parmesan

Day 6:
- Breakfast: Hummus and Vegetable Breakfast Bowl
- Lunch: Moroccan Lamb Stew
- Dinner: Lamb Shank Braised in Red Wine

Day 7:
- Breakfast: Maple Glazed Carrot Muffins
- Lunch: Chicken and Broccoli Alfredo
- Dinner: Roasted Lamb with Rosemary and Garlic

Week 5

Day 1:
- Breakfast: Mango and Lime Quinoa Salad
- Lunch: Grilled Pigeon with Mediterranean Vegetables
- Dinner: Beef and Mushroom Stroganoff

Day 2:
- Breakfast: Protein-Packed Breakfast Bars
- Lunch: Split Pea Soup
- Dinner: Fisherman's Stew

Day 3:
- Breakfast: Pumpkin Spice Smoothie
- Lunch: White Bean and Kale Stew
- Dinner: Chicken Fajitas

Day 4:
- Breakfast: Spinach and Feta Omelette
- Lunch: BBQ Chicken Pizza
- Dinner: Seafood Chowder

Day 5:
- Breakfast: Chicken Sausage and Sweet Potato Hash
- Lunch: Lamb Biryani
- Dinner: Beef Tenderloin with Roasted Vegetables

Day 6:
- Breakfast: Salted Peanut Butter Oatmeal
- Lunch: Asian Chicken Salad
- Dinner: Braised Rabbit with Garlic and Rosemary

Day 7:
- Breakfast: Buckwheat Pancakes
- Lunch: Cornish Hen with Wild Rice Stuffing
- Dinner: Smoked Duck Salad with Pomegranate

Week 6

Day 1:
- Breakfast: Raspberry Almond Muffins
- Lunch: Herb-Crusted Haddock
- Dinner: Chicken Paella

Day 2:
- Breakfast: Tofu Scramble
- Lunch: Beef and Spinach Lasagna
- Dinner: Lamb Tagine with Apricots

Day 3:
- Breakfast: Baked Pears with Walnuts and Honey
- Lunch: Chicken and Vegetable Stir-Fry
- Dinner: Spiced Lentil and Rice Porridge

Day 4:
- Breakfast: Pumpkin Spice Smoothie
- Lunch: Turkey Stir-Fry with Cashews
- Dinner: Shrimp Scampi with Zucchini Noodles

Day 5:
- Breakfast: Quinoa Porridge
- Lunch: Grilled Pigeon with Mediterranean Vegetables
- Dinner: Chicken Piccata with Capers

Day 6:
- Breakfast: Spinach and Feta Omelette
- Lunch: Spicy Tuna Poke Bowl
- Dinner: Braised Rabbit with Garlic and Rosemary

Day 7:
- Breakfast: Chicken Sausage and Sweet Potato Hash
- Lunch: Buffalo Chicken Wrap
- Dinner: Cornish Hen with Wild Rice Stuffing

Week 7

Day 1:
- Breakfast: Salted Peanut Butter Oatmeal
- Lunch: Fisherman's Stew
- Dinner: Game Hen Stew with Barley

Day 2:
- Breakfast: Egg Muffins
- Lunch: White Bean and Kale Stew
- Dinner: Duck Breast with Orange Sauce

Day 3:

- Breakfast: Greek Yogurt Parfait
- Lunch: Chicken and Broccoli Alfredo
- Dinner: Grilled Beef Skewers

Day 4:

- Breakfast: Banana Oatmeal Pancakes
- Lunch: Lamb Shank Braised in Red Wine
- Dinner: Classic Beef Stew

Day 5:

- Breakfast: Hummus and Vegetable Breakfast Bowl
- Lunch: Chicken Taco Salad
- Dinner: Moroccan Chicken Tagine

Day 6:

- Breakfast: Mango and Lime Quinoa Salad
- Lunch: Beef and Barley Soup
- Dinner: Seafood Chowder

Day 7:

- Breakfast: Protein-Packed Breakfast Bars
- Lunch: Grilled Salmon with Lemon and Herbs
- Dinner: Turkey Meatballs in Tomato Basil Sauce

Week 8

Day 1:

- Breakfast: Almond Butter and Banana Sandwich
- Lunch: Smoked Duck Salad with Pomegranate
- Dinner: Roasted Partridge with Pear

Day 2:

- Breakfast: Kale and Potato Breakfast Hash
- Lunch: Minestrone Soup
- Dinner: Moroccan Lamb Stew

Day 3:

- Breakfast: Buckwheat Pancakes
- Lunch: Chicken Fajitas
- Dinner: Spiced Beef Patties

Day 4:

- Breakfast: Raspberry Almond Muffins
- Lunch: Grilled Octopus with Olives and Oregano
- Dinner: Beef Tenderloin with Roasted Vegetables

Day 5:
- Breakfast: Tofu Scramble
- Lunch: Turkey and Vegetable Soup
- Dinner: Split Pea Soup

Day 6:
- Breakfast: Baked Pears with Walnuts and Honey
- Lunch: Asian Chicken Salad
- Dinner: Turkey Taco Salad

Day 7:
- Breakfast: Pumpkin Spice Smoothie
- Lunch: Baked Turkey and Spinach Meatballs
- Dinner: Potato Leek Soup

Week 9

Day 1:
- Breakfast: Quinoa Porridge
- Lunch: Fisherman's Stew
- Dinner: Slow Cooker Pot Roast

Day 2:
- Breakfast: Spinach and Feta Omelette
- Lunch: Buffalo Chicken Wrap
- Dinner: Beef Gyros

Day 3:
- Breakfast: Chicken Sausage and Sweet Potato Hash
- Lunch: Moroccan Lamb Stew
- Dinner: Lamb and Spinach Lasagna

Day 4:
- Breakfast: Salted Peanut Butter Oatmeal
- Lunch: Grilled Pigeon with Mediterranean Vegetables
- Dinner: Spiced Lentil and Rice Porridge

Day 5:
- Breakfast: Egg Muffins
- Lunch: White Bean and Kale Stew
- Dinner: Chicken Piccata with Capers

Day 6:
- Breakfast: Greek Yogurt Parfait
- Lunch: Shrimp Scampi with Zucchini Noodles
- Dinner: Grilled Beef Skewers

Day 7:

- Breakfast: Banana Oatmeal Pancakes
- Lunch: Turkey Stir-Fry with Cashews
- Dinner: Braised Rabbit with Garlic and Rosemary

Week 10

Day 1:

- Breakfast: Hummus and Vegetable Breakfast Bowl
- Lunch: Chicken and Broccoli Alfredo
- Dinner: Game Hen Stew with Barley

Day 2:

- Breakfast: Mango and Lime Quinoa Salad
- Lunch: Spicy Tuna Poke Bowl
- Dinner: Duck Breast with Orange Sauce

Day 3:

- Breakfast: Protein-Packed Breakfast Bars
- Lunch: Minestrone Soup
- Dinner: Moroccan Chicken Tagine

Day 4:

- Breakfast: Almond Butter and Banana Sandwich
- Lunch: Grilled Salmon with Lemon and Herbs
- Dinner: Beef and Mushroom Stroganoff

Day 5:

- Breakfast: Kale and Potato Breakfast Hash
- Lunch: Grilled Octopus with Olives and Oregano
- Dinner: Moroccan Lamb Stew

Day 6:

- Breakfast: Buckwheat Pancakes
- Lunch: Fisherman's Stew
- Dinner: Slow Cooker Pot Roast

Day 7:

- Breakfast: Raspberry Almond Muffins
- Lunch: Turkey and Vegetable Soup
- Dinner: Beef Gyros

WEEKLY MEAL PLANNER + WORKBOOK

	BREAKFAST	LUNCH	DINNER	SNACKS
MONDAY				
TUESDAY				
WEDNESDAY				
THURSDAY				
FRIDAY				
SATURDAY				
SUNDAY				

What are your top three health goals you hope to achieve by following the POTS diet?

WEEKLY MEAL PLANNER + WORKBOOK

	BREAKFAST	LUNCH	DINNER	SNACKS
MONDAY				
TUESDAY				
WEDNESDAY				
THURSDAY				
FRIDAY				
SATURDAY				
SUNDAY				

Can you list your most frequent POTS symptoms? How severe are they on a scale from 1 to 10?

WEEKLY MEAL PLANNER + WORKBOOK

	BREAKFAST	LUNCH	DINNER	SNACKS
MONDAY				
TUESDAY				
WEDNESDAY				
THURSDAY				
FRIDAY				
SATURDAY				
SUNDAY				

Describe your current daily eating habits. What are the common foods and meal times?

WEEKLY MEAL PLANNER + WORKBOOK

	BREAKFAST	LUNCH	DINNER	SNACKS
MONDAY				
TUESDAY				
WEDNESDAY				
THURSDAY				
FRIDAY				
SATURDAY				
SUNDAY				

How much water do you typically drink in a day? Do you consume other fluids?

WEEKLY MEAL PLANNER + WORKBOOK

	BREAKFAST	LUNCH	DINNER	SNACKS
MONDAY				
TUESDAY				
WEDNESDAY				
THURSDAY				
FRIDAY				
SATURDAY				
SUNDAY				

Have you been advised to increase your salt intake? If so, how do you plan to incorporate more salt into your diet?

WEEKLY MEAL PLANNER + WORKBOOK

	BREAKFAST	LUNCH	DINNER	SNACKS
MONDAY				
TUESDAY				
WEDNESDAY				
THURSDAY				
FRIDAY				
SATURDAY				
SUNDAY				

Are there any foods you are allergic to or find difficult to digest?

WEEKLY MEAL PLANNER + WORKBOOK

	BREAKFAST	LUNCH	DINNER	SNACKS
MONDAY				
TUESDAY				
WEDNESDAY				
THURSDAY				
FRIDAY				
SATURDAY				
SUNDAY				

How often do you plan your meals in advance? How can you integrate meal planning into your routine?

WEEKLY MEAL PLANNER + WORKBOOK

	BREAKFAST	LUNCH	DINNER	SNACKS
MONDAY				
TUESDAY				
WEDNESDAY				
THURSDAY				
FRIDAY				
SATURDAY				
SUNDAY				

What is your comfort level with cooking? Do you feel confident preparing the recipes in the POTS diet plan?

WEEKLY MEAL PLANNER + WORKBOOK

	BREAKFAST	LUNCH	DINNER	SNACKS
MONDAY				
TUESDAY				
WEDNESDAY				
THURSDAY				
FRIDAY				
SATURDAY				
SUNDAY				

Who can support you as you make dietary changes? How can they assist you?

WEEKLY MEAL PLANNER + WORKBOOK

	BREAKFAST	LUNCH	DINNER	SNACKS
MONDAY				
TUESDAY				
WEDNESDAY				
THURSDAY				
FRIDAY				
SATURDAY				
SUNDAY				

How do you plan to track your symptoms and progress while following the POTS diet?

WEEKLY MEAL PLANNER + WORKBOOK

	BREAKFAST	LUNCH	DINNER	SNACKS
MONDAY				
TUESDAY				
WEDNESDAY				
THURSDAY				
FRIDAY				
SATURDAY				
SUNDAY				

How do you usually do your grocery shopping? Do you anticipate any challenges in finding POTS-friendly foods?

WEEKLY MEAL PLANNER + WORKBOOK

	BREAKFAST	LUNCH	DINNER	SNACKS
MONDAY				
TUESDAY				
WEDNESDAY				
THURSDAY				
FRIDAY				
SATURDAY				
SUNDAY				

How often do you eat out or order takeout? How can you make POTS-friendly choices when dining out?

WEEKLY MEAL PLANNER + WORKBOOK

	BREAKFAST	LUNCH	DINNER	SNACKS
MONDAY				
TUESDAY				
WEDNESDAY				
THURSDAY				
FRIDAY				
SATURDAY				
SUNDAY				

Have you noticed any patterns with meal timing and symptom severity? How can you adjust your meal times for better symptom management?

WEEKLY MEAL PLANNER + WORKBOOK

	BREAKFAST	LUNCH	DINNER	SNACKS
MONDAY				
TUESDAY				
WEDNESDAY				
THURSDAY				
FRIDAY				
SATURDAY				
SUNDAY				

Where do you see yourself in six months after following the POTS diet? What positive changes do you hope to experience?

Scan the QR code below to get a surprise bonus!